Arthritis

*How You Can Benefit from Diet,
Vitamins, Minerals, Herbs, Exercise,
and Other Natural Methods*

Arthritis

How You Can Benefit from Diet, Vitamins, Minerals, Herbs, Exercise, and Other Natural Methods

Michael T. Murray, N.D.

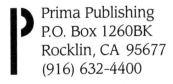 Prima Publishing
P.O. Box 1260BK
Rocklin, CA 95677
(916) 632-4400

Library of Congress Cataloging-in-Publication Data

Murray, Michael T.
    Arthritis : how you can benefit from diet, vitamins, minerals,
herbs, exercise, and other natural methods / Michael T. Murray.
        p.   cm. — (Getting well naturally series)
    Includes bibliographical references and index.
    ISBN 1-55958-491-2
    1. Arthritis—Alternative treatment.   2. Arthritis—Diet therapy.
I. Title.   II. Series.
    RC933.M87   1994
    616.7'2206—dc20

                                                                93–50095
                                                                CIP

    95 96 97 98 **AA**   10 9 8 7 6 5
Printed in the United States of America

Contents

Preface

Osteoarthritis, gout, and rheumatoid arthritis are three of the most common forms of arthritis. Each type has unique features, but there are some common features. More and more information is accumulating that indicates that diet plays a major role in the development, as well as the treatment and prevention, of all these forms of arthritis. In addition, evidence is showing that current medical treatment may be doing more harm than good.

The primary drugs used in the treatment of both osteoarthritis and rheumatoid arthritis are nonsteroidal anti-inflammatory drugs, or NSAIDs, a category that includes aspirin. Although these drugs are extensively used in the United States and may produce short-term benefit, research is indicating that in the treatment of osteoarthritis and rheumatoid arthritis, these drugs may be accelerating joint destruction and causing more problems down the road. Results of numerous studies have raised some interesting questions: Does medical intervention in some way promote disease progression? Can nutrition and various natural therapies enhance the body's own response and return to health? The information presented in this book shows clearly that the answer to both of these questions is yes.

In most cases, the natural approach provides far greater relief than does medical intervention, because the natural approach addresses the underlying disease process. The obvious question is this: If the natural approach is so effective, why aren't more doctors using it? There are some simple answers to this question. A doctor knows only what he or she has been taught. Since the typical medical doctor has less than 4 hours of training in nutrition, that doctor knows very little about how diet might influence arthritis. In fact, the majority of medical schools in the United States do not even require a course in nutrition.

Another reason why doctors are unaware of the natural approach to arthritis is the influence of the drug industry. In addition to the 45,000 drug company sales representatives who provide the majority of drug information to doctors, the drug companies control what is taught at medical schools and in continuing education programs. A recent editorial in a major medical journal discussed the influence of the drug industry on medical practice:[1]

> The overall influence of the industry is to emphasize drug treatment at the expense of other modalities: psychotherapy, social approaches, nutritional, herbal, and natural remedies, rehabilitation, general hygienic measures, nonpatentable drugs, or other alternative approaches. It focuses attention on disorders that are treatable by drugs, and may promote overdiagnosis. It reinforces the practice of dealing with disease by treatment of symptoms, and diverts interest from prevention.

Many doctors are beginning to recognize that their treatments are not providing the long-term benefit they had hoped to observe. In the treatment of arthritis, they see their patients continuing to suffer with their disease despite the fact the doctors are prescribing stronger and stronger medications. The doctors also see their patients experiencing side effects due to the drugs. More and more doctors are asking themselves: Am I really helping the patient?

Fortunately, there is an alternative approach to dealing with arthritis. It is my hope that the readers of this book will follow the recommendations given and experience relief from their arthritis without the use of drugs or surgery. I also hope that readers will share their experiences with others, including their physicians, so that even more people can benefit.

Acknowledgments

The major blessings in my life are my family and friends. My love for them truly makes life worth living.

Special appreciation to my wife, Gina, for being the answer to so many of my dreams; to my parents, Cliff and Patty Murray, and my grandmother, Pauline Shier, for a strong foundation and a lifetime of good memories; to Bob and Kathy Bunton for their love and acceptance; to Ben Dominitz and everyone at Prima for their commitment and support of my work; to Terry Lemerond and everyone at Enzymatic Therapy for all of their friendship and support over the years; and to Joseph Pizzorno and the students and faculty at Bastyr College who have given me encouragement and support. And finally, I am eternally grateful to all the researchers, physicians, and scientists who over the years have strived to better understand the use of natural medicines. Without their work, this series would not exist, and medical progress would halt.

Michael T. Murray, N.D.
January, 1994

Before You Read On

- Do not self-diagnose. Proper medical care is critical to good health. If you have symptoms suggestive of an illness, please consult a physician—preferably a naturopath, holistic physician or osteopath, chiropractor, or other natural health care specialist.

- If you are currently taking a prescription medication, you absolutely must consult your doctor before discontinuing it.

- If you wish to try the natural approach, discuss it with your physician. Since he or she is most likely unaware of the natural alternatives available, you may need to do some educating. Bring this book along with you to the doctor's office. The natural alternatives being recommended are based upon published studies in medical journals. Key references are provided if your physician wants additional information.

- Remember, although many natural alternatives, such as nutritional supplements and plant-based medicines, are effective on their own, they work even better if they are part of a comprehensive natural treatment plan that focuses on diet and lifestyle.

Osteoarthritis

1

What Is Osteoarthritis?

The most common form of arthritis is osteoarthritis, which is also known as degenerative joint disease. Osteoarthritis is seen primarily, but not exclusively, in the elderly. Surveys have indicated that over 40 million Americans have osteoarthritis, including 80% of persons over the age of 50. Under the age of 45, osteoarthritis is much more common in men; after age 45, it is more common in women than men.

The weight-bearing joints and joints of the hands are the joints most often affected by the degenerative changes associated with osteoarthritis. Specifically, extensive cartilage destruction is followed by cartilage hardening and the formation of large bone spurs in the joint margins. Cartilage serves an important role in joint function. Its gel-like nature provides protection to the ends of joints by acting as a shock absorber. Degeneration of the cartilage is the hallmark of osteoarthritis. With this degeneration comes inflammation, pain, deformity, and diminished range of motion in the joint.

Diagnostic Summary

- Mild early-morning stiffness, stiffness following periods of rest, pain that worsens on joint use, and loss of joint function
- Local tenderness, soft-tissue swelling, creaking and cracking of joints on movement, bony swelling, restricted mobility and other signs of degenerative loss of joint cartilage

Signs and Symptoms of Osteoarthritis

The onset of osteoarthritis can be very subtle. Morning joint stiffness is often the first symptom. As the disease progresses, there is pain on motion of the involved joint—pain that is worse after prolonged activity and relieved by rest. There is usually no sign of inflammation.

The specific clinical picture varies with the joint involved. Disease of the hands leads to pain and limitation of use. Knee involvement produces pain, swelling, and instability. Osteoarthritis of the hip causes local pain and a limp. Spinal osteoarthritis is very common and may result in compression of nerves and blood vessels, causing pain and vascular insufficiency.

The classic presentation of osteoarthritis is easy to distinguish from other types of arthritis—especially rheumatoid arthritis, which is usually associated with significant inflammation of surrounding soft tissue.

What Causes Osteoarthritis?

Osteoarthritis is divided into two categories, primary and secondary osteoarthritis. In primary osteoarthritis, the degenerative wear-and-tear process of aging usually starts to manifest as joint pain and stiffness at 50 to 60 years of age. In primary osteoarthritis, there is no apparent predisposing abnormality, such as previous injury. The cumulative effects of decades of use lead to the degenerative changes by stressing the integrity of the cartilage. Damage to the cartilage results in an uneven surface where joints meet. If the degeneration is severe enough, it can result in bone rubbing against bone.

One of the major reasons for the degeneration of cartilage is decreased ability to restore and manufacture normal cartilage structures. As we age, the number as well as the activity of important repair enzymes is greatly reduced, making the joint structures especially prone to damage. Therefore, as we age, we are more susceptible to primary osteoarthritis.

Secondary osteoarthritis is associated with some predisposing factor responsible for the degenerative changes. Some of the common predisposing factors include inherited abnormalities in joint structure or function; trauma (fractures along joint surfaces, surgery, and the like); presence of abnormal cartilage; and previous inflammatory disease of the joint, such as rheumatoid arthritis or gout.

The Natural Course of Osteoarthritis

Little is known concerning the natural course of osteo-arthritis—that is, the course of the disease if no treatment is given. However, data collected from the earliest signs of osteoarthritis to the most advanced stages suggest that cellular and tissue response is purposeful and is aimed at repair of the damaged joint structure. In other words, the body is striving to heal itself. The degenerative process contributing to osteoarthritis appears stoppable and, sometimes, reversible.[1] Therefore, the major goal of therapy should be to enhance the repair processes within the joints. Unfortunately, current medical treatment does not accomplish this goal and may actually inhibit joint repair.

There are a few studies that have attempted to determine the natural course of osteoarthritis.[1,2] In one study of patients with advanced osteoarthritis, researchers reported remarkable clinical improvement and X-ray films confirmed recovery of the joint space in 14 of 31 hips over a ten-year period.[2] The authors of the study purposely applied no therapy and regarded their results as reflecting the natural course of the disease. On the basis of results like these, some doctors and researchers are wondering if medical intervention can actually encourage the debilitating effects of osteoarthritis.

Current Medical Treatment of Osteoarthritis

The first drug generally used in the treatment of osteoarthritis and rheumatoid arthritis is aspirin. Aspirin is a nonsteroidal anti-inflammatory drug, or NSAID. Aspirin is often quite effective in relieving both the pain and inflammation. It is also relatively inexpensive. However, since the therapeutic dose required is relatively high (2 to 4 grams per day), toxicity often occurs. Tinnitus (ringing in the ears) and gastric irritation are early manifestations of toxicity.

Other NSAIDs are often used as well, especially when aspirin is ineffective or intolerable. The following are representative of this class of drugs:

Fenoprofen (Nalfon)
Ibuprofen (Motrin, Advil, Nuprin)
Indomethacin (Indocin, Indometh)
Meclofenamate (Meclofen, Meclomen)
Naproxen (Naprosyn)

Piroxicam (Feldene)

Sulindac (Clinoril)

Tolmetin (Tolectin)

Although these drugs have not proven to be more effective than aspirin, some may be better tolerated. However, they are also much more expensive than aspirin and still carry with them significant risk for side effects. They are, therefore, recommended only for short periods of time. In addition to being used for arthritis, NSAIDs are also used for headaches, low back pain, traumatic injury, postoperative pain, and menstrual cramps.

How NSAIDs work has not been completely established, but they are known to reduce inflammation by suppressing the formation of prostaglandins and related compounds, chemicals involved in the production of inflammation and pain.

Side Effects of NSAIDs

Since the dosage of NSAIDs necessary to suppress symptoms is usually quite high, so is the rate of side effects. The most common side effect of aspirin and other NSAIDs is damage to the intestinal tract and ulcer formation. NSAID-induced peptic ulcers can be serious and life threatening.

In addition to causing ulcers, NSAIDs often cause allergic reactions, easy bleeding and bruising, ringing in the ears, and fluid retention. More serious complications include kidney and liver damage.

NSAIDs in Arthritis: More Harm Than Good?

One side effect of aspirin and other NSAIDs that is not often mentioned is inhibition of cartilage repair (that is, inhibition of collagen matrix synthesis) and acceleration of cartilage destruction.[3,4] Since osteoarthritis is caused by degeneration of cartilage, NSAIDs may worsen the condition by inhibiting cartilage formation and accelerating cartilage destruction. Indeed, some clinical studies have shown that the use of NSAIDs is associated with acceleration of osteoarthritis and increased joint destruction.[5-7] The higher the dosage and the longer the use of NSAIDs, the greater the joint destruction.

Simply stated, *aspirin and other NSAIDs appear to suppress the symptoms but accelerate the progression of osteoarthritis.* Avoid using these drugs!

Final Comments

The current treatment of osteoarthritis needs to be evaluated according to three time-tested medical principles:

Principle 1. The healing power of nature: The human body has considerable power to heal itself. The role of the physician or treatment is to facilitate and enhance this process. The current medical treatment of osteoarthritis does not support the healing process.

Principle 2. First do no harm: As Hippocrates said, "Above all else, do no harm." The current treatment of osteo-arthritis seems to do more harm than good.

Principle 3. Identify and treat the cause: Of vital impor-tance is the treatment of the underlying causes of a dis-ease rather than suppression of the symptoms. The current drug treatment of osteoarthritis only suppresses symptoms. Because the drugs do not address the causes, the disease process progresses.

It is obvious that the current medical treatment of osteo-arthritis is less than ideal. Fortunately, an effective natural treatment is available—a treatment that can withstand scrutiny based on the three main principles of healing. The next chapter will discuss this treatment.

2

The Natural Approach
to Osteoarthritis

The natural approach to osteoarthritis seeks to address the factors responsible for joint degeneration. This approach primarily involves supporting normal cartilage function and repair. As stated in the previous chapter, research tells us that in osteoarthritis the body is striving to heal itself. The degenerative process contributing to osteoarthritis seems to be stoppable and, sometimes, reversible. Nutrition can play a major role in the prevention and treatment of osteoarthritis. Nutrition accomplishes the major goal of therapy: the enhancement of the repair processes within the joints.

Dietary Factors in Osteoarthritis

The dietary guidelines given in Chapter 7 provide the framework for the prevention and treatment of osteoarthritis. It is critical that the diet be rich in fruits and vegetables— rich sources of natural plant compounds that can protect against cellular damage, including damage to joints. The cells throughout the human body are constantly under attack. The culprits are compounds known as free radicals and pro-oxidants. These highly reactive molecules can bind to and destroy cellular components. Free radical damage is what makes us age. Free radical damage is also linked to osteoarthritis and the development of many other problems: cancer, heart disease, cataracts, Alzheimer's disease, and virtually every other chronic degenerative disease.

Although the body creates free radicals during metabolism, the environment contributes greatly to an individual's free radical load. Cigarette smoking, for example, greatly increases the free radical load. Many of the harmful effects of smoking are related to the extremely high levels of free radicals being inhaled. These compounds deplete key antioxidant nutrients, such as vitamin C and beta-carotene. Other external sources of free radicals include sunlight, X rays, air pollutants, pesticides, anesthetics, aromatic hydrocarbons, fried food, solvents, alcohol, and formaldehyde. These greatly stress the body's antioxidant mechanisms.

Human enzymes and antioxidants from the plant foods we consume can protect against harm from free radicals and oxidative damage. The helpful substances in these foods include carotenes, flavonoids, vitamins C and E, and sulfur-containing compounds. Free radical–scavenging enzymes— catalase, superoxide dismutase, and glutathione peroxidase —can break down the free radicals before the radicals react with molecules in the cells. Taking the enzymes orally is of limited value; oral supplementation with these enzymes has not been shown to increase tissue levels or offer any real benefit. However, ingesting antioxidant nutrients (such as manganese, sulfur-containing amino acids, carotenes, flavonoids, and vitamin C) can increase tissue concentrations of the enzymes.

The other way in which the cell can protect itself against free radical, or oxidative, damage is via chemical neutralization. In this process, antioxidants bind to, or neutralize, the free radical or pro-oxidant. For example, the nutritional antioxidants—vitamins C and E, beta-carotene, and selenium—block free radical damage by reacting chemically with the free radical or pro-oxidant to neutralize it. Ingesting rich sources of these compounds from fresh uncooked fruits and vegetables can increase tissue concentrations of these nutrients, thereby supporting normal protective mechanisms in the cells. One of the easiest and most efficient ways to increase your intake of these foods is to drink homemade fresh fruit and vegetable juices. If you have arthritis or if you just want to be healthier, get a juicer and use it regularly.

Beneficial Foods

Some specific foods especially beneficial in the treatment of all forms of arthritis are flavonoid-rich fruits, such as cherries, blueberries, and blackberries (see Chapter 4). Also important are sulfur-containing foods, such as garlic, onions, Brussels sprouts, and cabbage. The sulfur content in the fingernails of arthritis sufferers is lower than that in the fingernails of healthy controls.[1] Normalizing the sulfur content by administering intravenous or intramuscular colloidal sulfur alleviated pain and swelling, according to clinical data from the 1930s.[2] Presumably, increasing the sulfur content of the body by increasing consumption of sulfur-rich foods or by taking nutritional supplements containing sulfur (supplements such as glucosamine sulfate, discussed in a moment) may be of similar benefit.

Possible Negative Effects of Nightshade-Family Vegetables

A number of specific diets have been recommended in the treatment of osteoarthritis. The most popular is the one recommended by Norman Childers, Ph.D. His diet is founded on a personal experience. Childers eliminated foods from the genus *Solanaceae* (nightshade family) from his own diet and found that this simple dietary elimination cured his osteo-arthritis.[3] Childers developed a theory that genetically susceptible individuals might develop arthritis, as well as a variety of other complaints, from long-term low-level consumption of the alkaloids found in tomatoes, potatoes, eggplant, peppers, and tobacco. Presumably, these alkaloids inhibit normal cartilage repair in the joints or promote the inflammatory degeneration of the joint. To test his theory, Dr. Childers conducted an informal study of over 5,000 arthritis patients who agreed to avoid eating nightshade-family vegetables. Over 70% reported relief from aches and pains. Although a strict scientific study has not confirmed the beneficial effect of the Childers approach, the diet may offer some benefit to certain individuals. It is certainly worth a try.

Nutritional Supplements in Osteoarthritis Treatment

Although the dietary recommendations already mentioned are often quite therapeutic on their own, nutritional supplementation can provide additional help for those with osteoarthritis. Of particular importance is supplying additional antioxidant nutrients (selenium, manganese, and vitamins C and E) and the nutrients important in the manufacture of joint substances. Of these, niacinamide, pantothenic acid, vitamin B6, and zinc are especially important. But, before we look at these nutrients, the first substance I want to discuss is glucosamine. It is a classic example of how a natural substance improves a condition by addressing the underlying cause and supporting the body's ability to heal itself.

Glucosamine Sulfate

Glucosamine is a naturally occurring substance found in high concentrations in joint structures. When taken as a nutritional supplement, glucosamine sulfate appears to be nature's best remedy for osteoarthritis. In the body, the main action of glucosamine on joints is to stimulate the manufacture of cartilage components. In other words, glucosamine is responsible for stimulating the manufacture of substances necessary for joint repair.

It appears that, as people age, they lose the ability to manufacture sufficient levels of glucosamine. The result is that cartilage loses its ability to hold water and act as a shock absorber. The inability to manufacture glucosamine has been suggested as the major factor leading to osteoarthritis. This link led researchers in Europe to ask an important question: What would happen if individuals with osteoarthritis took glucosamine? The results have been astonishing.

In relieving the pain and inflammation of osteoarthritis, numerous double-blind studies have shown glucosamine sulfate to produce much better results than NSAIDs and placebos. These results occur despite the fact that glucosamine sulfate exhibits very little direct anti-inflammatory effect and no direct analgesic, or pain-relieving, effect.[4–9] NSAIDs offer purely symptomatic relief and may actually promote the disease process; glucosamine sulfate addresses the cause of osteoarthritis. By getting at the root of the problem, glucosamine sulfate not only improves the symptoms, including pain, it also helps the body repair damaged joints. This effect is outstanding, especially when safety and lack of side effects are considered. The side effects and risks associated with NSAIDs currently used in the treatment of osteoarthritis are significant. The therapeutic margin, a measure of safety, is 10 to 30 times more favorable for glucosamine sulfate than for commonly used NSAIDs.[10]

The beneficial results of glucosamine are more obvious the longer it is used. Because glucosamine sulfate is not an anti-inflammatory or pain-relieving drug, it takes a while to produce results. But once it starts working, it will produce much better results than NSAIDs. For example, in one study that compared glucosamine sulfate to ibuprofen (Motrin),

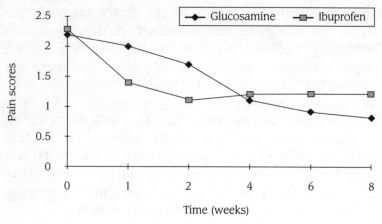

Figure 2.1   Glucosamine versus ibuprofen

pain scores decreased faster in the first two weeks in the ibuprofen group. However, by week 4 the group receiving the glucosamine sulfate was doing significantly better than the ibuprofen group.[9] Figure 2.1 presents these pain scores in the form of a graph.

Glucosamine sulfate products are available at health food stores or through nutritional-oriented physicians. Be sure to use glucosamine sulfate versus glucosamine hydrochloride or N-acetylglucosamine—the scientific studies were performed with the sulfate form. The standard dose for glucosamine sulfate is 500 milligrams, three times per day. As mentioned earlier, the body tolerates glucosamine sulfate extremely well. In addition, there are no contraindications or adverse interactions with drugs. Glucosamine sulfate may cause some gastrointestinal upset (nausea, heartburn, and the like) in rare instances. If this occurs, try taking it with meals.

Cartilage Extracts

Cartilage extracts—including purified chondroitin sulfate, sea cucumber, green-lipped mussel, and shark cartilage—are popular nutritional supplements that may help those with osteoarthritis by improving cartilage function. Compared to glucosamine sulfate, the degree of purity and effectiveness of these compounds varies widely.

Shark cartilage, sea cucumber, and green-lipped mussel contain several molecules known as glycosaminoglycans (GAGs), or mucopolysaccharides. One of the key GAGs is chondroitin sulfate. Chondroitin sulfate is composed of repeating units of glucosamine sulfate with attached sugar molecules. The difference between glucosamine sulfate, cartilage extracts, and chondroitin sulfate products is similar to the difference between crude ore (shark cartilage or chondroitin sulfate) and pure gold (glucosamine). Although there is gold in crude ore, if you are trying to make jewelry, you would do better to use the pure gold. If you are trying to restore cartilage and joint structures, it is best to use glucosamine sulfate rather than chondroitin sulfate or shark cartilage.

Why? The major reason is the ease with which glucosamine sulfate can be absorbed. Cartilage extracts; shark cartilage; and green-lipped mussel, sea cucumber, and chondroitin sulfate products are composed of large molecules that are extremely difficult to absorb. The absorption rate for chondroitin sulfate, the smallest molecule in these products, is estimated to be between 0% and 8%.[11] In contrast, 98% of orally administered glucosamine sulfate is absorbed intact.[12] Since chondroitin sulfate is 200 times larger than glucosamine sulfate, the difference in absorption is similar to the difference between swallowing a whole watermelon (chondroitin sulfate) and swallowing a sesame seed (glucosamine sulfate).

After glucosamine sulfate is absorbed, it is preferentially taken up by cartilage and other joint structures, where it stimulates the manufacture of chondroitin sulfate and other mucopolysaccharides.

From a clinical perspective, glucosamine is extremely effective if given orally. In contrast, in osteoarthritis treatment the effectiveness of oral chondroitin sulfate, green-lipped mussel, sea cucumber, and shark cartilage is a subject of considerable debate. Most of the positive clinical studies with glycosaminoglycan preparations have utilized injectable forms.[11,13] Pharmaceutical-grade cartilage preparations and chondroitin sulfate injections, used according to established protocols, have well-documented benefit. Unfortunately, this therapy is currently not available in the United States. What about the benefit of orally administered chondroitin sulfate; cartilage extracts; and green-lipped mussel, sea cucumber, and shark cartilage? Based on existing scientific literature, it is unlikely these products are effective in treating either osteoarthritis or rheumatoid arthritis.[11,14] If any benefit is derived from these products, it is most likely due to the freeing of glucosamine.

When all is considered, it is quite easy to see why glucosamine sulfate is preferred to cartilage extracts in the treatment of osteoarthritis.

Vitamins C and E

Vitamin C and vitamin E have been shown to exert some beneficial effects in the treatment of osteoarthritis.[15] Both nutrients are important antioxidant substances, which help prevent damage to cartilage components.

Vitamin C is critically involved in the manufacture of collagen, the major support protein of cartilage. Without sufficient levels of vitamin C in the joint tissues, collagen synthesis halts. Deficient vitamin C intake is common in the elderly and is known to result in altered collagen synthesis and compromised joint tissue repair.[16] Low vitamin C levels may be a major factor in some patients with osteoarthritis.

Experimental evidence indicates that the higher the vitamin C level, the greater the protection against osteoarthritis.[17] A study of osteoarthritis in guinea pigs showed that cartilage erosion and changes in and around an osteoarthritic joint were less pronounced in animals taking high doses of vitamin C.[15]

The debate over how much vitamin C is required by humans is ongoing. At one end of the spectrum, two-time Nobel Prize winner Linus Pauling and his followers recommend an intake somewhere between 2 to 9 grams a day during periods of health. During times of stress or illness, they say, intake should be higher. At the other end of the spectrum, the recommended dietary allowance (RDA) for vitamin C has been established at 60 milligrams for adults. I lean toward Pauling's recommendation. My recommendation to patients with osteoarthritis is that they supplement their diet with 1,000 to 3,000 milligrams of vitamin C each day. But I want to stress that you should not rely on supplements to meet all your vitamin C requirements. Vitamin C–rich foods are also rich in compounds like flavonoids and carotenes, which work to enhance the effects of vitamin C as well as exert favorable effects of their own.

Vitamin E supplementation also appears to be indicated. In one clinical trial, osteoarthritis patients used 600 IU (international units) of vitamin E per day. The benefit of the vitamin E was significant and was thought to be due to the antioxidant and membrane-stabilizing actions of the vitamin.[15] Subsequent studies have shown that vitamin E has an ability to inhibit the breakdown of cartilage as well as stimulate increased manufacture of cartilage components such as glycosaminoglycans.[18]

Although both vitamin C and vitamin E exert beneficial effects when taken individually, taking them in combination may provide even better results. One research study concluded:[15]

> Thus, both vitamins E and C appear to enhance the stability of the complex structure comprising cartilage. Judicious use of these vitamins in the treatment of osteoarthritis, either alone or in combination with other therapeutic means, may thus be of great benefit to the patient population by retarding the erosion of cartilage.

Niacinamide *medical supervision*

Niacinamide is a form of vitamin B3. Dr. William Kaufman and others have reported that vitamin B3 produces very good clinical results in the treatment of osteoarthritis.[19,20] Using a high dose of niacinamide (900 to 4,000 milligrams in divided daily doses), Dr. Kaufman has treated hundreds of patients with osteoarthritis or rheumatoid arthritis. Although niacinamide is better tolerated than niacin, another form of vitamin B3, high doses of niacinamide can result in some side effects, including liver damage. Therefore, it is a good idea to utilize this natural treatment under <u>medical supervision,</u> especially when more than 900 milligrams of niacinamide is taken each day.[14,15] A simple blood test for liver function every three months is all that is necessary for proper monitoring.

Pantothenic Acid

Pantothenic acid, or vitamin B5, supplementation may be of benefit for patients with osteoarthritis. Acute deficiency of pantothenic acid in the rat causes a pronounced failure of cartilage growth and eventually produces lesions similar to those caused by osteoarthritis. The implication is that a low pantothenic acid level is a factor in the development of human osteoarthritis. The administration of 12.5 milligrams of pantothenic acid per day has been shown to produce some benefit for patients with osteoarthritis.[21,22] However, a larger, better-controlled study failed to show any real benefit with pantothenic acid, even when the dosage was increased to 2 grams daily.[23] Since most multiple-vitamin, multiple-mineral formulas provide at least 12.5 milligrams of pantothenic acid, additional supplementation doesn't appear necessary, given its questionable benefit.

Vitamins A, B6, and E; Zinc, Boron, and Copper

These nutrients are required for the synthesis of normal collagen and maintenance of cartilage structures. A deficiency of any one of these would allow accelerated joint degeneration. Adequate intake of these nutrients can be achieved by taking a quality multiple-vitamin, multiple-mineral formula that provides at least the RDA for these nutrients. Boron may not be included in some multiple-vitamin, multiple-mineral formulas, because no RDA for boron has been established. If the formula you take does not contain boron, take a supplement that provides you with 6 to 9 milligrams daily.

Typically, the standard American diet is severely deficient in fruits and vegetables, the major food sources of boron. Hence, many Americans' intake of boron is insufficient. However, since the level of boron in foods is directly related to the level of boron in the soil, simply eating more fruits and vegetables may not be enough. Studies from a number of different countries have found that the lower the level of boron in the soil, the more often people develop osteoarthritis.

Boron supplementation has been used in the treatment of osteoarthritis in Germany since the mid 1970s. This use was recently evaluated in a small double-blind clinical study. Of the patients receiving 6 milligrams of boron (as sodium tetraborate decahydrate), 71% improved; only 10% in the placebo group improved.[24] The preliminary indication is that boron supplements are of value in osteoarthritis treatment.

Plant-Based Medicines in Osteoarthritis Treatment

Many plants have been used in the treatment of osteoarthritis. If inflammation is present, botanicals and nutritional agents possessing anti-inflammatory activity are indicated. As inflammation is more of a factor in rheumatoid arthritis, natural anti-inflammatory substances are discussed in Chapter 6. Particularly useful are extracts of curcumin (a component of turmeric) and ginger.

In most cases of osteoarthritis, plant-based treatment addresses the underlying factors responsible for the degeneration. For example, plants rich in substances known as phytoestrogens are often used. These plant compounds are capable of binding to estrogen receptors on cartilage cells, thereby preventing the binding of the body's own estrogen to the receptor. The higher prevalence of osteoarthritis in women suggests that estrogens may play a role. Experimental studies have demonstrated that estrogen promotes osteoarthritis.[25] Several botanicals that have historically been used in the treatment of osteoarthritis are licorice root (*Glycyrrhiza glabra*), dong quai (*Angelica sinensis*), and alfalfa (*Medicago sativa*). Apparently, they work by effectively blocking the negative effects of estrogen in osteoarthritis.

Although phytoestrogen-containing herbs are of value in treating osteoarthritis, perhaps the best way to increase their intake is to increase the intake of food that contains them. Food sources of phytoestrogens include fennel, celery, parsley, soy, nuts, whole grains, and apples. These foods, along with the regular consumption of alfalfa sprouts and licorice tea, will provide a much higher level of phytoestrogens than taking small amounts of herbs. Of course, if you are a menopausal woman, phytoestrogen herbs can be of tremendous benefit in dealing with the symptoms of menopause. If you are going through menopause, I strongly encourage you to read *Menopause,* another book in the Getting Well Naturally series (Prima Publishing, Rocklin, CA, 1994).

Boswellia

Another plant historically used in the treatment of osteoarthritis is *Boswellia serrata,* a large branching tree native to India. Boswellia yields an exudative gum resin known as salai guggul. Although salai guggul has been used for centuries, newer preparations concentrated for the active components (boswellic acids) are giving better results.

Boswellic acid extracts have demonstrated anti-arthritic effects in a variety of animal studies. There are several mechanisms of action, including inhibition of inflammatory mediators, prevention of decreased glycosaminoglycan synthesis, and improved blood supply to joint tissues.[26,27] Clinical studies using plant-based formulas containing boswellia have yielded good results in osteoarthritis as well as rheumatoid arthritis treatment.[28] The standard dosage for boswellic acids in arthritis is 400 milligrams, three times daily. No side effects due to boswellic acids have been reported.

Devil's Claw

A plant native to Africa, devil's claw (*Harpagophytum procumbens*) has a long history of use in the treatment of arthritis. Scientific studies of inflammation in animals show that devil's claw causes an anti-inflammatory and analgesic effect comparable to that of the potent drug phenylbutazone.[29] Several clinical studies have also demonstrated some benefit. However, other studies have indicated that devil's claw has little, if any, anti-inflammatory activity.[30,31]

The equivocal research results may reflect the mechanism of action of devil's claw, which is inconsistent with that of current anti-inflammatory drugs, or it could reflect a lack of quality control (standardization) of the devil's claw preparations used. Until these questions are answered, other natural measures should be used before trying devil's claw in the treatment of osteoarthritis. At this time, devil's claw appears to be better suited in the treatment of gout (see Chapter 4). Nonetheless, here are the recommendations in regard to devil's claw.

Dosage (take these amounts, three times daily)

Dried powdered root	1 to 2 grams or as a cup of tea
Tincture (1:5)	4 to 6 milliliters (1 to 1½ teaspoons)
Dry solid extract (3:1)	400 milligrams

Physical Therapy in Osteoarthritis Treatment

Various physical therapy treatments—exercise, heat, cold, diathermy, and ultrasound—performed by physical therapists, naturopathic physicians, and chiropractors are often very beneficial in improving joint mobility and reducing pain for sufferers of osteoarthritis. The importance of physical therapy appears to be quite significant, especially when administered regularly. Much of the benefit of physical therapy is thought to be a result of achieving the proper water content within the joint capsule, thereby facilitating the elimination of waste products and utilization of nutrients. Combining physical therapy measures—such as short-wave diathermy therapy with periodic ice massage, rest, and appropriate exercises—appears to be the most sensible approach.

Proper exercises include isometric exercises and swimming. These increase circulation to the joint and strengthen surrounding muscles without placing too much strain on the joint.

Final Comments

Although the primary treatment of osteoarthritis should consist of dietary therapy, nutritional and plant-based supplements can also be of exceptional value. Let me try and give some clear recommendations in terms of where to start with nutritional and plant-based supplements for osteoarthritis.

1. Take a high-potency multiple-vitamin, multiple-mineral supplement that provides at least 100% of the RDA for all nutrients.
2. Take an antioxidant supplement that will provide higher-than-RDA levels of some of the nutritional antioxidants, including vitamins C and E.

3. Take glucosamine sulfate at a dose of 500 milligrams, three times daily.

Although further support is rarely necessary, the additional nutritional and plant-based supplements discussed in this chapter can be used if needed. Because the natural measures, such as glucosamine sulfate, may take up to a month or two to produce their benefit, some patients with severe osteoarthritis may need to continue with their NSAIDs. In this case, it is imperative to employ measures to protect the gastrointestinal tract from damage. Perhaps the best single recommendation is to use a special extract of licorice known as DGL, which is short for deglycyrrhizinated licorice. DGL has been shown to reduce the gastric bleeding caused by aspirin and other NSAIDs. DGL is strongly indicated for patients requiring long-term treatment with ulcer-causing drugs, such as NSAIDs and corticosteroids.[32]

A history of NSAID or corticosteroid use is associated with peptic ulcers. Numerous studies over the years have found DGL to be an effective anti-ulcer compound. DGL's mode of action is different than that of the current medications used for the treatment of peptic ulcers. Rather than inhibit the release of acid, licorice stimulates the normal defense mechanisms that prevent ulcer formation. Specifically, DGL improves both the quality and quantity of the protective substances that line the intestinal tract, increases the lifespan of the intestinal cell, and improves blood supply to the intestinal lining.

DGL is superior to popular prescription drugs for ulcers. In several head-to-head comparison studies, DGL has been shown to be more effective than Tagamet, Zantac, or antacids in both short-term treatment of peptic ulcers and in consequent maintenance therapy.[33,34] In addition, the drugs studied are associated with significant side effects, but DGL is extremely safe and is only a fraction of the cost. For example, Tagamet or Zantac typically costs well over $100 for a month's supply. A month's supply of DGL is available in health food stores for $15.

To be effective in healing or prevention, it appears that DGL must mix with saliva. DGL may promote the release of salivary compounds that stimulate the growth and regeneration of stomach and intestinal cells. The standard daily dose for DGL, in 380-milligram chewable tablets, is 2 to 4 tablets between, or 20 minutes before, meals. Continue using DGL for 8 to 16 weeks after stopping NSAID use. The DGL will help heal the damaged intestinal tract.

Gout

3

What Is Gout?

Gout is a common type of arthritis. It is caused by an increased concentration of uric acid in biological fluids. Uric acid is the final breakdown product of purine metabolism. Purines are made in the body and are also ingested in foods. In gout, uric acid crystals are deposited in joints, tendons, kidneys, and other tissues, where they cause considerable inflammation and damage.

Gout is associated with affluence and is often called the rich man's disease. Throughout history, the sufferer of gout has been depicted as a portly, middle-aged man sitting in a comfortable chair, with one foot resting painfully on a soft cushion as he consumes great quantities of meat and wine. In fact, the traditional picture does have some basis in reality: Meats, particularly organ meats, are high-purine foods, and alcohol inhibits the kidneys from ridding themselves of uric acid. Furthermore, even today, gout is primarily a disease of adult men. Over 95% of sufferers of gout are men over the age of 30. The incidence of gout is approximately 3 adults in

1,000, although as many as 10% to 20% of the adult population have elevated uric acid levels in the blood.

Diagnostic Summary
- Acute onset of intense joint pain typically involving the first joint of the big toe (about 50% of cases)
- Elevated uric acid level in the blood
- Periods without symptoms between acute attacks
- Identification of urate crystals in joint fluid
- Aggregated deposits of urate crystals in and around the joints of the extremities, but also in subcutaneous tissue, bone, cartilage, and other tissues
- Uric acid kidney stones
- Familial disease; affects males more often than females (95% of the time)

Signs and Symptoms of Gout

The first attack of gout is characterized by intense pain, usually involving only one joint. The first joint of the big toe is affected in nearly half the first attacks and is at some time involved in over 90% of gout cases. If the attack progresses, fever and chills appear. The first attacks usually occur at night and are usually preceded by a specific event, such as dietary excess, alcohol ingestion, trauma, certain drugs, or surgery.

The classic description of gout was by an English physician, Sydenham, who suffered from gout in 1683.[1] Little has changed in the clinical picture of gout in over three hundred years.

The victim goes to bed and sleeps in good health.
About two o'clock in the morning he is awakened
by a severe pain in the great toe; more rarely in
the heel, ankle, or instep. The pain is like that of a

dislocation, and yet parts feel as if cold water were poured over them. Then follows chills and shivers, and a little fever. The pain which at first was moderate, becomes more intense. With its intensity the chills and fever increase. After a time this comes to a height, accommodating itself to the bones and ligaments of the tarsus and metatarsus. Now it is a violent stretching and tearing of the ligaments—now it is a gnawing pain and now a pressure and tightening. So exquisite and lively meanwhile is the feeling of the part affected, that it cannot bear the weight of bedclothes nor the jar of a person walking in the room. The night is passed in torture, sleeplessness, turning the part affected, and perpetual change of posture; the tossing about of the body being as incessant as the pain of the tortured joint, and being worse as the fit comes on. Hence the vain effort by change of posture, both in the body and the limb affected, to obtain an abatement of pain.

Subsequent attacks are common, with the majority having another attack within one year. However, nearly 7% never have a second attack. Chronic gout is extremely rare, due to the advent of dietary therapy and drugs that lower uric acid levels. Some degree of kidney dysfunction occurs in nearly 90% of subjects with gout, and there is a higher risk of kidney stones.

What Causes Gout?

Gout is classified into two major categories: primary and secondary. Primary gout accounts for about 90% of all cases; secondary gout accounts for only 10%. The cause of primary gout is usually unknown. There are, however, several genetic defects in which the exact cause of the elevated uric acid is known.

The increased level of uric acid in the blood that is a characteristic of primary gout is due to one of three causes: (1) increased synthesis of uric acid (the cause of most cases of gout), (2) reduced ability to excrete uric acid (the cause of about 30% of gout cases), and (3) overproduction of uric acid as well as underexcretion of uric acid (the cause of very few cases). Although the exact metabolic defect that engenders gout is not known in the majority of cases, gout is one of the most controllable metabolic diseases (see Figure 3.1).

Secondary gout refers to those cases in which the elevated uric acid level is secondary to some other disorder, such as excessive breakdown of cells or some form of kidney disease. Diuretic therapy for high blood pressure and low-dose aspirin therapy are also important causes of secondary gout. Both these therapies decrease uric acid excretion.

An adult male excretes 200 to 600 milligrams of uric acid daily, in the urine. This amount is two-thirds of what is excreted; the rest is in the bile and other gastrointestinal tract secretions. The dietary component of uric acid in the blood is usually only 10% to 20% of the total uric acid. For an individual with significant uric acid in the blood, however, enough dietary uric acid can increase crystal formation in tissues.

Almost all the uric acid in the blood is filtered in the kidney: Only the small amount bound to protein is not filtered. Excretion into the urine is peculiar in that about 80% of the filtered uric acid is reabsorbed.

Uric acid is a highly insoluble molecule. At pH 7.4 and body temperature, the serum is saturated at 6.4 to 7.0 milligrams per 100 milliliters. Although higher concentrations do not necessarily result in deposition of uric acid crystals (some unknown factor in the blood appears to inhibit crystal precipitation), the chance of an acute attack is greater than 90%

Metabolic Dysfunction

Increased production of purines (primary)
   Idiopathic (unknown)
   Specific enzyme defects (e.g., Lesch-Nyhan syndrome, glycogen storage disease, etc.)

Increased production of purines (secondary)
   Increased turnover of purines
      Cancer
      Chronic hemolytic anemia
      Cytotoxic drugs
      Psoriasis
   Increased synthesis (e.g., glucose-6-phosphatase deficiency)
   Increased breakdown of purines
      Fructose ingestion or infusion
      Exercise

Kidney Dysfunction

Decreased kidney clearance of uric acid (primary)
   Intrinsic kidney disease

Decreased kidney clearance of uric acid (secondary)
   Functional impairment of tubular secretion
      Drug-induced (e.g., as a result of thiazides, probenecid, salicylates, ethambutol, pyrazinamide)
      Hyperlacticemia (e.g., lactic acidosis, alcoholism, toxemia of pregnancy, chronic beryllium disease)
      Hyperketoacidemia (e.g., diabetic ketoacidosis, diabetes insipidus)
      Bartter's syndrome
      Chronic lead intoxication
      Glucose-6-phosphatase deficiency

Figure 3.1   Causes of gout

when the level is above 9 milligrams per 100 milliliters. Lower temperatures decrease the saturation point of uric acid, which may explain why urate deposits tend to form in areas such as the top of the ear, where the temperature is lower than the mean body temperature. Uric acid is insoluble below pH 6.0 and can precipitate as the urine is concentrated in the collecting ducts and passed to the bladder (see Tables 3.1 and 3.2).

Table 3.1   Prevalence of Gouty Arthritis by Maximum Uric Acid

Serum Urate	Percentage Afflicted	
(mg/100 ml)	Men	Women
<6	0.60%	0.08%
6.0–6.9	1.9	3.3
7.0–7.9	16.7	17.4
8.0–8.9	25.0	0.0
9+	90.0	0.0

Table 3.2   Solubility of Uric Acid as a Function of Temperature

Temperature (degrees C)	Maximum Solubility (mg/100 ml)
37	6.8
35	6.0
30	4.5
25	3.3
20	2.5
15	1.8
10	1.2

Current Medical Treatment of Gout

There are basically two types of gout medications: drugs used to treat acute attacks of gout and drugs that reduce the level of uric acid in the body. In the treatment of acute attacks, doctors prescribe colchicine or nonsteroidal anti-inflammatory drugs (NSAIDs), such as indomethacin, phenyl-butazone, naproxen, or fenoprofen. Colchicine is the drug of choice when the diagnosis of gout is in question. NSAIDs are now preferred over colchicine in acute attacks where a firm diagnosis of gout has been made.[2] Since NSAIDs are discussed fully elsewhere (see page 6), only colchicine will be discussed here.

In the treatment of chronic gout, physicians often measure the amount of uric acid in a 24-hour collection of urine to identify whether a patient is an overproducer of uric acid (greater than 800 milligrams) or an underexcretor (less than 800 milligrams). The overproducer is usually prescribed allopurinol; the underexcretor, probenecid or sulfinpyrazone.

Colchicine

Colchicine is an anti-inflammatory drug that was originally isolated from the meadow saffron plant (*Colchicum autumnale*). Colchicine has no effect on uric acid levels. Rather, it stops the inflammatory process by lowering the acidity of the joint tissues, thereby increasing the solubility of uric acid and dissolving uric acid crystals. Colchicine also inhibits the migration of white blood cells into areas of inflammation.

Colchicine is still the preferred drug when the diagnosis of gout is in question. If the cause is gout, colchicine will bring about almost immediate relief. If it isn't gout, colchicine will not be effective. It is somewhat diagnostic in initial attacks, because over 90% of patients with gout show dramatic improvement in symptoms within the first 12 hours after receiving colchicine. However, as many as 80% of patients are unable to tolerate an optimal dose because of gastrointestinal side effects: severe nausea, abdominal cramps, vomiting, or diarrhea. These side effects may precede or coincide with clinical improvement.

As this chapter will discuss later, low doses of colchicine are often used with probenecid to prevent recurrent gout attacks. Products that contain this combination include Colabid, ColBENEMID, and Proben-C.

Colchicine is an extremely powerful drug that has significant side effects. Side effects are typically a function of dosage—that is, the greater the dosage, the more likely it is that side effects will appear. As mentioned, most patients will experience significant gastrointestinal discomfort. Other possible side effects include allergic reactions; loss of hair; suppression of bone marrow, resulting in low white blood cell counts, anemia, abnormal bleeding and bruising, and fatigue; peripheral nerve inflammation characterized by numbness, "pins and needles" sensations, pain, and weakness in the hands or feet; liver damage; and inflammation of the colon, resulting in bloody diarrhea.

Allopurinol

Allopurinol lowers uric acid levels by inhibiting its formation. It does this by inhibiting the activity of xanthine oxidase, the enzyme responsible for the final conversion of purines into uric acid. Allopurinol is best used in treating gout patients that overproduce, as opposed to underexcrete, uric acid.

In general, allopurinol is well tolerated. The most common side effect is a skin rash. Because these skin reactions can be quite severe, and even fatal, treatment with allopurinol must be discontinued immediately if a rash develops. Other possible side effects include headache, dizziness, fatigue, loss of hair, and liver damage.

Probenecid and Sulfinpyrazone

These two drugs increase the excretion of uric acid. They are used primarily in the long-term management of gout in patients who, because of inability to excrete uric acid, have elevated levels of uric acid in blood and tissue.

Because probenecid and sulfinpyrazone increase the excretion of uric acid, they increase the risk of developing kidney stones. Patients with a history of kidney stones or kidney disease should not take either drug.

Other than kidney stones, the most common side effects of probenecid and sulfinpyrazone are gastrointestinal irritation (nausea, vomiting, gastric pain, and the like), headache, and mild skin rashes. Other possible side effects include reduced appetite, sore gums, liver damage, bone marrow suppression, and kidney damage.

Final Comments

It is a well-accepted fact that most cases of gout can be treated effectively with diet alone. However, with the advent of modern drug therapy, many physicians do not stress the value of diet therapy to their patients. It is far easier to simply prescribe a pill than to educate the patient about more healthful food choices. Given the side effects of the drugs and the safety and effectiveness of dietary therapy, the failure of physicians to discuss dietary therapy with their patients is a great disservice.

4

The Natural Approach
to Gout

I n concept, the natural approach to chronic gout does not differ substantially from the standard medical approach. However, rather than using drugs to keep uric acid levels within the norm, natural measures are employed. Foremost in the natural approach is diet. The dietary treatment of gout involves the following guidelines:

Elimination of alcohol intake

Low-purine diet

Achievement of ideal body weight

Liberal consumption of complex carbohydrates

Low fat intake

Low protein intake

Liberal fluid intake

Increased consumption of flavonoids

Alcohol

Alcohol increases uric acid production. It reduces uric acid excretion by increasing lactate production (a result of the breakdown of alcohol), which impairs kidney function. The net effect is a significant increase in serum uric acid levels—that is, the levels of uric acid in the blood. This explains why alcohol consumption is often a precipitating factor in acute attacks of gout. For many individuals, elimination of alcohol is all that is needed to reduce uric acid levels and prevent gout.[1]

Low-Purine Diet

A low-purine diet has been the mainstay of the dietary therapy for gout for many years. Foods with high purine levels should be entirely omitted. These include organ meat, meat, shellfish, yeast (brewer's and baker's), herring, sardines, mackerel, and anchovies.

Weight Reduction

Individuals with gout are typically obese, prone to high blood pressure and diabetes, and are at a greater risk for cardio-vascular disease. Weight reduction of obese individuals significantly reduces serum uric acid levels. Achieving ideal body weight may be the most important dietary goal in gout treatment.

Carbohydrates, Fats, and Protein

Refined carbohydrates and saturated fats should be kept to a minimum. The former increase uric acid production; the latter decrease uric acid excretion. Protein intake should not be excessive—it has been shown that uric acid synthesis may be accelerated in both normal and gouty patients by a high protein intake.

Fluid Intake

Liberal fluid intake keeps the urine dilute and promotes the excretion of uric acid. Furthermore, dilution of the urine reduces the risk of kidney stones.

Flavonoids

Consuming the equivalent of ½ pound of fresh cherries per day has been shown to be very effective in lowering uric acid levels and preventing attacks of gout.[2] Cherries, hawthorn berries, blueberries, and other dark red–blue berries are rich sources of anthocyanidins and proanthocyanidins. These flavonoid compounds are what give these fruits their deep red–blue color. They are also the compounds that make these fruits remarkable in their ability to prevent destruction of joint structures. The importance of flavonoids in preventing the destruction of collagen is discussed in Chapter 6.

Nutritional Supplements in the Treatment of Gout

Since diet alone is effective in treating most cases of gout, specific nutritional supplements for gout are usually not necessary. In fact, high doses of vitamin C or niacin may actually raise uric acid levels. A general recommendation for sufferers of gout is to simply take a quality multiple-vitamin, multiple-mineral formula that provides 100% of the RDAs. If additional nutritional support is needed, quercetin, omega-3 oils, and folic acid can be used.

Quercetin

The flavonoid quercetin has demonstrated several effects in experimental studies that indicate its possible benefit to individuals with gout. Quercetin inhibits uric acid production in a similar fashion to the drug allopurinol. In addition, quercetin inhibits the manufacture and release of inflammatory compounds.[3,4] Quercetin is widely found in fruits and vegetables. In the treatment of gout, nutritional supplementation can provide higher amounts than diet alone. For best results, 200 to 400 milligrams of quercetin should be taken with bromelain (see Chapter 6) between meals, three times daily. Bromelain may help enhance the absorption of quercetin as well as exert anti-inflammatory effects of its own.

Omega-3 Oils

Omega-3 oils, like flaxseed oil and fish oils, limit the production of compounds known as leukotrienes, which are the major mediators of inflammation and tissue damage in gout. (A complete discussion of the omega-3 oils is provided in Chapter 6.) The same recommendations given for the treatment of rheumatoid arthritis are appropriate in the treatment of gout.

Folic Acid

Folic acid has been shown to inhibit xanthine oxidase, the enzyme responsible for producing uric acid.[5] In fact, research has demonstrated that a derivative of folic acid is an even greater inhibitor of xanthinoxidase than allopurinol, suggesting that folic acid at pharmacological doses may be an effective treatment in gout. Positive results in the treatment of gout have been reported, but the data are incomplete and the accompanying research was without adequate controls.[6] The dosage of folic acid required is in the range of 10 to 40 milligrams per day.

Folic acid has been used at these high dosages with no reported toxicity and is certainly safer than current drugs used in treating gout. However, there have been reports of high-dose folic acid interfering with some drugs used to treat epilepsy. High doses of folic acid may also mask the symptoms of a vitamin B12 deficiency. Because of these concerns, undertake folic acid therapy only under the supervision of a physician.

Plant-Based Medicines in Gout Treatment

Plant-based medicines are usually not necessary in the treatment of gout. However, in the initial stages of dietary therapy, clinical research in Europe appears to indicate that devil's claw (see Chapter 2) may be of benefit. In addition to relieving joint pain, clinical trials found that devil's claw reduced serum cholesterol and uric acid levels.[7]

Saturnine Gout

Lead toxicity can cause a secondary type of gout, sometimes called saturnine gout.[8] Historically, saturnine gout was due to the consumption of alcoholic beverages stored in containers containing lead (for example, lead crystal). This is still a concern, but nowadays lead contamination from the environment (water, air, food, and so on) is a bigger problem. In the United States alone, lead from industrial sources and leaded gasoline contribute more than 600,000 tons of lead, which is dumped into the atmosphere to be inhaled or—after being deposited on food crops, in fresh water, or soil—to be ingested. Hair mineral analysis is a good screening test for lead toxicity. I recommend it be performed in any patient suffering from gout.

If lead is the source of the problem, particular foods and nutrients can help "get the lead out." These include artichokes, beets, carrots, dandelion, cabbage-family vegetables, whole grains, legumes, vitamin C, zinc, choline, methionine, cysteine, and flavonoids.

Rheumatoid Arthritis

5

What Is Rheumatoid Arthritis?

R heumatoid arthritis is a chronic inflammatory condition that affects the entire body but especially the synovial membranes of the joints. It is a classic example of an auto-immune disease, a condition in which the body's immune system attacks the body's own tissue. Other autoimmune diseases that can lead to arthritis include ankylosing spondylitis, systemic lupus, and scleroderma.

In rheumatoid arthritis, the joints typically involved are the hands and feet, wrists, ankles, and knees. Involved joints are characteristically quite warm, tender, and swollen. The skin over the joint takes on a ruddy purplish hue. As the disease progresses, joint deformities result in the hands and feet. Terms used to describe these deformities include *swan neck, boutonniere,* and *cockup toes.*[1,2]

Somewhere between 1% and 3% of the population is affected; female patients outnumber males almost 3:1; and the usual age of onset is 20 to 40 years, although rheumatoid arthritis may begin at any age.

Diagnostic Summary

- Fatigue, low-grade fever, weakness, joint stiffness, and vague joint pain may proceed the appearance of painful, swollen joints by several weeks.
- Severe joint pain, with much inflammation, begins in small joints, but progressively affects all joints in the body.
- X-ray findings usually show soft-tissue swelling, erosion of cartilage, and joint-space narrowing.
- Rheumatoid factor (RF) is present in the blood.
- Systemic manifestations are common. These include inflammation of the blood vessels (vasculitis), muscle wasting, skin nodules, inflammation of the heart and lungs, enlargement of the spleen, anemia, and depressed white blood cell counts.

Rheumatoid arthritis is easily recognized in its most advanced and characteristic form. However, diagnosis of early rheumatoid arthritis is often much more difficult. If you feel you may have rheumatoid arthritis, visit your physician for definitive diagnosis.

Signs and Symptoms of Rheumatoid Arthritis

The onset of rheumatoid arthritis is usually gradual, but occasionally it is quite abrupt. Fatigue, low-grade fever, weakness, joint stiffness, and vague joint pain appear first. Several weeks later joints become painful and swollen. Several joints are usually involved in the onset, typically in a symmetrical fashion—that is, both hands, wrists, or ankles. In about one-third of persons with rheumatoid arthritis, initial involvement is confined to one or a few joints.

Most persons with rheumatoid arthritis feel fatigued as a result of the anemia that usually accompanies the disease.

Other common accompanying problems include carpal tunnel syndrome (tingling and pain in the fingers, caused by pressure on the nerve as it enters the hand through the wrist) and Raynaud's phenomenon (a condition where the blood flow through the fingers is severely reduced when they are exposed to cold).

In some cases, soft nodules develop beneath the skin over bony surfaces. More serious complications, such as inflammation of the heart and lungs, are usually only seen in severe cases.

What Causes Rheumatoid Arthritis?

There is abundant evidence that rheumatoid arthritis is an autoimmune reaction, where antibodies develop against components of joint tissues. Yet what triggers this auto-immune reaction remains largely unknown. Speculation and investigation has focused on genetic susceptibility, abnormal bowel permeability, and microorganisms, as well as dietary factors. In short, rheumatoid arthritis is a classic example of a multifactorial disease in which an assortment of genetic and environmental factors contribute to the disease process.

Genetic Factors

A specific genetic marker (histocompatibility antigen HLA-DRw4) is found in 70% of patients with rheumatoid arthritis; it is found in only 28% of the general population. This strongly implies that the likelihood of developing rheumatoid arthritis is influenced by genetic factors that govern immune re-sponse. In support of this theory is the fact that severe rheumatoid arthritis occurs at four times the average rate in children of parents with rheumatoid arthritis.

As strong as these genetic associations are, environmen-tal factors are necessary for the development of the disease.

This is perhaps most evident in studies of identical twins. These studies show that it is quite rare for both twins to develop rheumatoid arthritis.[1]

Abnormal Bowel Permeability

An interesting association between rheumatoid arthritis and abnormal bowel function may provide a unified theory of the cause of rheumatoid arthritis. What is currently known is that individuals with rheumatoid arthritis have increased intestinal permeability. This means that their intestines are too "leaky."[2,3] Food allergies (discussed in Chapter 7) are thought to contribute greatly to the increased permeability of the gut in rheumatoid arthritis. The release of histamine and other allergic compounds after eating an allergic food greatly increases the "leakiness" of the gut.

The result of a leaky gut is an increased absorption of large dietary and bacterial molecules. Normally, these molecules are too large to be absorbed. The body's response to these molecules is to form antibodies to bind them. Antibodies, released by white blood cells, bind to foreign molecules such as those found on bacteria, viruses, and cancer cells. When an antibody binds to the foreign molecule or antigen, the result is the formation of what is called an immune complex. An immune complex is composed of a large molecule, which is the antigen, and an antibody.

In the case of rheumatoid arthritis, food and bacterial molecules are acting as antigens that are being bound by antibodies. The resulting immune complex triggers the immune system to release compounds to destroy it. These compounds work great when antibodies bind to bacteria and viruses. When immune complexes are deposited in joint tissues, however, these compounds actually destroy not only the immune complex, but also the surrounding joint tissue.

The presence of immune complexes in joint tissue is one of the major factors contributing to the development of rheumatoid arthritis. The immune complexes result in much inflammation and joint destruction. As the joint tissues are being destroyed, large molecules normally protected from the immune system by cell membranes and connective tissue become exposed. The result is that the body develops antibodies to these exposed antigens.[4]

Another way in which the body may develop antibodies to its own tissue is by developing cross-reacting antibodies. The increased gut permeability and altered bacterial flora result in the absorption of antigens that are very similar to antigens in joint tissues. Antibodies formed to these antigens would cross-react with the antigens in the joint tissues. Increasing evidence supports this concept.

Clinically, physicians use the presence of immune complexes, which is called the rheumatoid factor (RF), to monitor rheumatoid arthritis patients. The blood and joint fluid of nearly all individuals with rheumatoid arthritis contain the RF. Most RF is formed in the affected joints by white blood cells. The level of RF can be measured and usually correlates with the severity of arthritis symptoms. That is, when the RF level is high, severity is high; when the RF level is low, severity is low.

Possible Microbial Causes

Many interesting hypotheses suggest that microorganisms are responsible for rheumatoid arthritis. As interesting as the various microbial hypotheses are, however, they are not in themselves comprehensive enough to explain all the events observed in rheumatoid arthritis. A variety of microorganisms (for example, Epstein–Barr virus, rubella virus, amoebic organisms, and mycoplasma) have been suggested as causative factors in the development of rheumatoid arthritis despite the fact that no microbial agent has been consistently isolated in rheumatoid arthritis patients.[5]

Microbial factors, particularly their role in increasing the level of circulating immune complexes, definitely contribute to the disease process of rheumatoid arthritis. At this time, though, it appears highly unlikely that there is a single causative microbe. Nonetheless, researchers continue to search for a causative agent.

To summarize, extensive research suggests that high levels of circulating immune complexes containing microbial antigens in general, as well as the increased microbial antigenic load observed in rheumatoid arthritis patients, are of greater significance than antibodies to one particular organism or group of organisms.

Current Medical Treatment of Rheumatoid Arthritis

Standard medical therapy is of limited value in most cases of rheumatoid arthritis. Current medical treatment fails to address the complexity of this disease in an appropriate manner. The treatment of rheumatoid arthritis primarily involves the use of aspirin and other nonsteroidal anti-inflammatory drugs, or NSAIDs (see Chapter 1). As in osteoarthritis, use of these drugs in the treatment of rheumatoid arthritis suppresses symptoms but accelerates factors that promote the disease process. In the case of rheumatoid arthritis, NSAIDs have been shown to greatly increase the already hyperpermeable gastrointestinal tract of rheumatoid arthritis sufferers.[6] The use of NSAIDs in rheumatoid arthritis is also a significant cause of serious gastrointestinal tract reactions, including ulcers, hemorrhage, and perforation. Due to NSAIDs use by individuals with rheumatoid arthritis, approximately 20,000 hospitalizations and 2,600 deaths occur each year.[7]

Corticosteroids are often used as an alternative or adjunct to NSAIDs in the treatment of rheumatoid arthritis. Most experts and medical textbooks clearly state that long-term use of corticosteroids for this purpose is not advised, because of side effects. Nonetheless, long-term corticosteroid use by patients with rheumatoid arthritis is quite common.

If NSAID and cortisone therapy does not offer benefit, more aggressive and potentially more toxic treatments are used along with continued use of NSAIDs and corticosteroids. Hydroxychloroquine, gold therapy, penicillamine, azathioprine, methotrexate, and cyclophosphamide are examples of drugs currently in use. Unfortunately, in most cases, the benefit produced by these drugs is greatly outweighed by significant toxicity. The use of these drugs often requires the use of additional drugs to deal with side effects. It is not uncommon for individuals with rheumatoid arthritis to be on 12 or more prescription drugs at one time. And finally, joint surgery and replacement are reserved for the most severe cases.

A Closer Look at Corticosteroids

Corticosteroids are a group of drugs that are similar in structure and function to the natural corticosteroid hormones produced by the adrenal glands. These drugs, like the natural hormones, can participate in a wide range of activities and are used in the treatment of a wide range of allergic and inflammatory conditions. In addition to rheumatoid arthritis, corticosteroids are used in the treatment of asthma; autoimmune disorders, such as multiple sclerosis and lupus; Crohn's disease; ulcerative colitis; and serious cases of psoriasis and eczema. The drugs are also used to suppress the immune system in selected types of cancers and in the prevention or rejection of a transplanted organ.

Prednisone is by far the most often prescribed oral corticosteroid. Other drugs in this category include prednisolone, methylprednisolone, dexamethasone, and betamethasone. Prednisone blocks many key steps in the allergic and inflammatory response, including the production and secretion, by white blood cells, of the so-called inflammatory mediators (histamine, prostaglandins, and leukotrienes). This disruption of the normal defense functions of the white blood cells is great at stopping the inflammatory response, but it essentially cripples the immune system.

Although prednisone is often of great benefit in the short-term management of many chronic inflammatory diseases, long-term use generally causes more problems than benefit. (The next section will discuss some of the side effects.) For this reason, most physicians of patients with rheumatoid arthritis try to reserve the use of prednisone for treatment of acute worsening.

Because long-term treatment with corticosteroids suppresses the natural production of the corticosteroids produced by the adrenal gland, sudden withdrawal of the drugs may lead to collapse, coma, and death. *Do not change your dosage of any corticosteroid without the supervision of a physician.*

The side effects of oral corticosteroids are a function of dosage levels and length of time on the medication. Most of the side effects are not due to taking too much of the drug for a short period of time, but rather reflect long-term use. At lower doses (less than 10 milligrams per day), the most notable side effects are usually increased appetite, weight gain, retention of salt and water, and increased susceptibility to infection. These side effects are almost always expected with corticosteroids.

Common side effects of long-term corticosteroid use at higher dosage levels include depression and other mental or emotional disturbances (up to 57% of patients being treated with high doses of prednisone for long periods of time develop these symptoms); high blood pressure; diabetes; peptic ulcers; acne; for women, excessive facial hair; insomnia; muscle cramps and weakness; thinning and weakening of the skin; osteoporosis; and susceptibility to the formation of blood clots.

A Closer Look at Disease-Modifying Drugs

Hydroxychloroquine, gold, penicillamine, azathioprine, methotrexate, and cyclophosphamide are drugs used to treat rheumatoid arthritis. They are often referred to as disease-modifying drugs. Here is a brief description of each of these agents, in their usual order of use.

Hydroxychloroquine A drug originally used in the treatment of malaria, hydroxychloroquine (Plaquenil) is also used in the treatment of rheumatoid arthritis. Researchers think it works by inhibiting the immune system. Since rheumatoid arthritis is an autoimmune disease, the drug effectively cripples the immune system from damaging the joint tissues.

Hydroxychloroquine must be used for at least six months to determine if it is going to be of value in the treatment of rheumatoid arthritis. Since hydroxychloroquine is associated with a high rate of side effects, use is often discontinued before this time period. Mild adverse effects include skin rashes, loss of hair, headache, blurring of vision, ringing in the ears, loss of appetite, nausea, vomiting, stomach cramps, and diarrhea. Severe side effects include emotional or psychotic mental changes; seizures; excessive muscle weakness; damage to the eyes, with significant impairment of vision; anemia; decreased white blood cell counts; and frequent infections.

Gold Salts Injection of gold salts aids about half the rheumatoid arthritis patients who receive them, but nearly one-third of these patients experience severe side effects. Oral gold salts are slightly less toxic than injections, but the treatment still causes skin rashes; painful mouth ulcers; bone marrow suppression; and, in some cases, even more serious side effects, such as kidney damage. Like hydroxychloroquine, a trial of six months is required to determine the benefit of therapy with gold salts.

Penicillamine   A drug used in the treatment of copper, mercury, and lead poisoning, penicillamine works by binding to these metals and promoting their excretion. Penicillamine has been used in the treatment of rheumatoid arthritis since the early 1960s. Its use has fallen out of favor in the 1990s, because of a growing concern about its safety as well as questions about its effectiveness. Penicillamine is a powerful drug that can cause kidney damage, blood and bone marrow toxicity, and severe muscular weakness. Like other disease-modifying drugs, it must be used for at least six months to determine if it is effective.

Azathioprine   This drug suppresses the immune system. It is often used to severely impair the immune system after organ transplantation, in an attempt to prevent tissue rejection. In rheumatoid arthritis, it is also used to block the immune system. Azathioprine is even more powerful than the previously discussed disease-modifying drugs, and it provides more immediate benefits. With this increased potency comes significant toxicity. Side effects include skin rash, loss of appetite, nausea, vomiting, diarrhea, sores on lips and mouth, bone marrow suppression, weakness, and fatigue. Azathioprine is also associated with an increased risk of certain cancers.

Methotrexate   Used primarily in the treatment of cancer and a severe disabling form of psoriasis, methotrexate works by inhibiting the utilization of the B vitamin folic acid, which is required for cell reproduction. Without the ability to utilize folic acid, cells are unable to divide and multiply. The goal of its use in the treatment of rheumatoid arthritis is to inhibit the replication of white blood cells. This inhibition results in suppression of the immune system. After azathioprine, methotrexate is the next step in potency and toxicity. Side effects include gastrointestinal ulceration and bleeding; loss of hair; mouth and throat ulcers; severe bone marrow suppression;

damage to the lungs, liver, and kidneys; increased rate of infections; and increased risk of cancer.

Cyclophosphamide This drug is used primarily in the treatment of various forms of cancer. It is even more powerful than all the previously described disease-modifying drugs. Toxicity is a major problem. The side effects of cyclophosphamide are comparable to those of methotrexate, but more severe.

Final Comments

There is little argument that rheumatoid arthritis is an aggressive disease that calls for aggressive measures. There is also little argument that current medical treatment of rheumatoid arthritis is aggressive. The big question is this: Is aggressive chemotherapy for rheumatoid arthritis actually providing benefit? Granted, the severe joint destruction of rheumatoid arthritis is being reduced—but at what cost to the patient?

Researchers are only beginning to determine the effects of treatment on the long-term outcome of rheumatoid arthritis. To fully answer the questions raised in the previous paragraph, many patients with rheumatoid arthritis must be followed for at least 20 years. Many of the disease-modifying drugs have only been used for the last two or three decades.

A study published in the British medical journal *The Lancet* evaluated the long-term outcome of therapy in 112 rheumatoid arthritis patients who were treated with conventional drug therapy.[8] After 20 years, despite aggressive therapy with standard drug regimens, only 18% of all patients were able to lead normal lives. Most patients (54%) were either dead or severely disabled (35% had died; 19% were severely disabled). Most mortalities were directly related to rheumatoid arthritis. The results of this study clearly indicate that, although current drug therapy may be effective in providing short-term benefit, this approach is not providing long-term benefits to patients with rheumatoid arthritis. Obviously, a better approach is needed. Such an approach is offered in the next chapter.

6

The Natural Approach to Rheumatoid Arthritis

M any factors contribute to rheumatoid arthritis. The natural approach involves reducing as many of these factors as possible, including poor digestion, food allergies, abnormal gut permeability, circulating immune complexes, and excessive inflammatory processes. Foremost in the natural approach is the use of diet to control inflammation.

Diet has been strongly implicated in rheumatoid arthritis for many years, both in regard to cause and cure. Population studies have demonstrated that rheumatoid arthritis is not found in societies that eat a more "primitive" diet and is found at a relatively high rate in societies consuming the so-called Western diet.[1] Therefore, a diet rich in whole foods, vegetables, and fiber and low in sugar, meat, refined carbohydrate, and saturated fat appears to offer some protection against developing rheumatoid arthritis. In addition, dietary therapy is showing tremendous promise in the treatment of rheumatoid arthritis.[2–4] The major focus in dietary therapy is eliminating food allergies, modifying the intake of dietary fats and oils, and increasing the intake of antioxidant nutrients.

Food Allergies and Rheumatoid Arthritis

Elimination of food allergens has been shown to offer significant benefit to some individuals with rheumatoid arthritis.[5-8]
Virtually any food can aggravate rheumatoid arthritis, but the
most common offending foods are wheat, corn, milk and
other dairy products, beef, and nightshade-family foods (tomato, potato, eggplant, peppers, and tobacco) as well as food
additives. Methods for determining food allergens are provided in Chapter 7.

A recent study highlights the effectiveness of eliminating
food allergens as part of a healthy diet and lifestyle program
in the treatment of rheumatoid arthritis.[9] In a 13-month study
conducted in Norway at the Oslo Rheumatism Hospital, two
groups of patients suffering from rheumatoid arthritis were
studied to determine the effect of diet on their condition. One
group followed a therapeutic diet (the treatment group); those
in the other group (the control group) were allowed to eat
as they wished. Both groups started the study by visiting a
"health farm," or what we in America call a spa, for four weeks.

The treatment group began the therapeutic diet by
fasting for 7 to 10 days. Dietary intake during the fast consisted of herbal teas; garlic; vegetable broth; decoction of
potatoes and parsley; and juices of carrots, beets, or celery.
Interestingly enough, no fruit juices were allowed. Patients
with rheumatoid arthritis have historically benefited from
fasting; however, strict water fasting should only be done
under direct medical supervision.[10-12] Fasting decreases the
absorption of food allergens as well as reduces the levels of
inflammatory mediators. A juice fast or a fast similar to the
one used in this study is safer than a water fast and may actually yield better results. Short-term fasts of three to five days
duration are recommended during acute worsening of rheumatoid arthritis.

After the fast the patients reintroduced a "new" food item
every second day. If they noticed an increase in pain, stiff-

ness, or joint swelling within 2 to 48 hours, they omitted the new item from the diet for at least seven days before reintroducing it a second time. If the food again caused worsening of symptoms, it was ommitted permanently from the diet.

The results of the study indicated that short-term fasting followed by a vegetarian diet resulted in "a substantial reduction in disease activity" in many patients. The results indicated a therapeutic benefit beyond elimination of food allergens alone. The authors suggested that the additional improvements were due to changes in dietary fatty acids. Before discussing the role dietary fats play in rheumatoid arthritis, let's examine the importance of proper digestion.

Digestion and Rheumatoid Arthritis

Proper digestion is a requirement for optimum health, and incomplete or disordered digestion can be a major contributor to the development of many diseases, including rheumatoid arthritis. The problem is not only that ingestion of foods and nutritional substances is of little benefit when breakdown and assimilation are inadequate, but also that incompletely digested food molecules can be inappropriately absorbed into the body. Since many individuals with rheumatoid arthritis are deficient in digestive factors (including hydrochloric acid and pancreatic enzymes), incomplete digestion may be a major factor in rheumatoid arthritis.[13,14]

Digestion occurs as a result of both physical and chemical processes. The physical changes of food are brought about by the grinding, crushing, and mixing of the food mass (chyme) with digestive juices during propulsion through the digestive tract. Chewing food thoroughly is the first aspect of good digestion. Chewing provides more than a mechanical effect; in addition, it mixes the food with saliva. Saliva contains an enzyme, salivary amylase (ptyalin), which breaks down starch molecules into smaller sugars.

It is the role of the esophagus to transport food and liquids from the mouth to the stomach. The stomach primarily functions in digestion of proteins and ionization of minerals. The stomach secretes hydrochloric acid, various hormones, and enzymes, and it activates the secretion of digestive enzymes by the pancreas, and bile by the gallbladder.

Many individuals with rheumatoid arthritis are deficient in hydrochloric acid. *Hypochlorhydria* refers to deficient gastric acid secretion; *achlorhydria* refers to a complete absence of gastric acid secretion. The best method of diagnosing a lack of gastric acid is a procedure known as the Heidelberg gastric analysis.[15] This technique utilizes an electronic capsule attached to a string. The patient swallows the capsule, which the string keeps in the stomach. The capsule measures the pH of the stomach and sends a radio message to a receiver, which then records the pH level. The response of the stomach to bicarbonate is the true test of the ability of the stomach to secrete acid.[16] After the test, the capsule is pulled up by the string.

Since not everyone can have Heidelberg gastric analysis to determine the need for gastric acid supplementation, another method of determination is often used. If an individual is experiencing any of the signs or symptoms of gastric acid insufficiency, which are listed in Figures 6.1 and 6.2, the method outlined in the next section can determine how much hydrochloric acid supplementation the patient needs.

Bloating, belching, burning, and flatulence immediately after meals

A sense of fullness after eating

Indigestion, diarrhea, or constipation

Multiple food allergies

Nausea after taking supplements

Itching around the rectum

Figure 6.1   Common symptoms of low gastric acidity

Weak, peeling, and cracked fingernails

Dilated blood vessels in the cheeks and nose

Acne

Iron deficiency

Chronic intestinal parasites or abnormal flora

Undigested food in stool

Chronic yeast (*Candida albicans*) infections

Upper digestive tract gassiness

Figure 6.2   Common signs of low gastric acidity

Protocol for Determining Hydrochloric Acid Dosage

Begin by taking 1 tablet or capsule containing 10 grains (600 milligrams) of hydrochloric acid at your next large meal. If this does not produce a warming sensation or abdominal discomfort, at every meal after that of the same size, take 1 more tablet or capsule than you did the time before. Continue to increase the dose until you reach 7 tablets or when you feel abdominal warmth or discomfort, whichever occurs first. A feeling of warmth in the stomach means that you have taken too many tablets for that meal and you need to take 1 less tablet for a meal of that size. It is a good idea to try the larger dose again, at another meal, to make sure that it was the hydrochloric acid that caused the warmth and not something else.

After you have found the largest dose that you can take at your large meals without feeling warmth or discomfort, maintain that dose at all meals of similar size. You will need to take fewer at smaller meals. When taking a number of tablets or capsules, take them throughout the meal.

As your stomach begins to regain the ability to produce the amount of hydrochloric acid needed to properly digest your food, you will notice the warm feeling again and will have to cut down the dose.

Pancreatic Enzymes and Rheumatoid Arthritis

The pancreas produces enzymatic secretions required for the digestion and absorption of food. Each day the pancreas secretes about 1.5 quarts of pancreatic juice in the small intestine. Enzymes secreted include lipases, which digest fat; proteases, which digest proteins; and amylases, which digest starch molecules.

Physicians use both physical symptoms and laboratory tests to assess pancreatic function. Common symptoms of pancreatic insufficiency include abdominal bloating and discomfort, gas, indigestion, and the passing of undigested food in the stool. For laboratory diagnosis, most nutrition-oriented physicians use comprehensive stool and digestive analysis. This comprehensive analysis can usually reveal the level of pancreatic enzymes being dumped into the intestines from the pancreas by determining the level of excess fat in the stool, excess nitrogen in the stool, and the presence of any other partially or completely undigested food elements. In addition, complete stool and digestive analysis can reveal the health of the bacterial flora, which often reflects the degree of pancreatic function.

Pancreatic enzyme products are prepared from fresh hog pancreas. Figure 6.3 lists the clinical uses of pancreatic enzymes. Pancreatic enzymes are most often employed in the treatment of impaired digestion; food allergies; and autoimmune diseases, such as rheumatoid arthritis.

Several human studies have shown that, when supplemental pancreatic protease or proteolytic enzymes, such as trypsin and chymotrypsin, are given orally, they are absorbed intact into the bloodstream in an enzymatically active form.[17,18] Even more dramatic is the finding that pancreatic enzymes are not only absorbed intact from the gut, but also transported through the bloodstream, taken up intact by pancreatic secretory cells, and resecreted into the

Digestive disturbances

Pancreatic insufficiency

Cystic fibrosis

Food allergies

Autoimmune disorders
    Rheumatoid arthritis
    Lupus
    Scleroderma
    Multiple sclerosis

Various cancers

Thrombophlebitis

Sports injuries and trauma

Viral infections
    Herpes zoster (shingles)
    AIDS

Figure 6.3   Clinical uses of pancreatic enzymes

intestines by the pancreas.[19] The existence of this circulation of proteolytic enzymes is quite similar to the recycling of bile salts by the liver.

The Importance of the Proteases

Although starch and fat digestion can be carried out satisfactorily without the help of pancreatic enzymes, the proteases are critical to proper protein digestion. Incomplete digestion of proteins creates a number of problems for the body, including the development of allergies and formation of toxic substances produced during putrefaction. *Putrefaction* refers to the breakdown of protein material by bacteria.

As well as being necessary for protein digestion, the proteases serve several other important functions. For example, the proteases, as well as other digestive secretions, are largely responsible for keeping the small intestine free from parasites (including bacteria, yeast, protozoa, and intestinal worms).[20] A lack of proteases or other digestive secretions greatly increases an individual's risk of having an intestinal infection, including an overgrowth of the yeast *Candida albicans.*

The proteases are also of benefit in treating food allergies. For a food molecule to produce an allergic response, it must be a fairly large molecule. In studies performed in the 1930s and '40s, pancreatic proteases were shown to be quite effective in treating food allergies.[21] Many practitioners are not aware of, or they have forgotten about, these early studies. Typically, individuals who do not secrete enough proteases suffer from multiple food allergies. It appears that many individuals with rheumatoid arthritis may secrete insufficient amounts of proteases.

The proteases are also important in preventing tissue damage during inflammation and stopping the formation of fibrin clots. Fibrin forms a wall around an inflamed area. The wall blocks blood and lymph vessels; this leads to swelling. Proteases cause an increase in the breakdown of fibrin, a process known as fibrinolysis. Fibrin can also cause the development of blood clots, which can become dislodged and produce strokes or heart attacks. Protease enzymes are often used in the treatment of thrombophlebitis, a disease in which blood clots develop in veins. The veins may become inflamed and a clot can dislodge, causing stroke or heart attack. Pancreatic enzymes and protease enzyme preparations have been shown to be useful in the treatment of many acute and chronic inflammatory conditions, including rheumatoid arthritis.[22–24]

Another benefit of the proteases in the treatment of rheumatoid arthritis is the prevention of the deposit of immune complexes in body tissues. Diseases associated with high levels of circulating immune complexes include rheumatoid arthritis, lupus erythematosus, periarteritis nodosa, scleroderma, ulcerative colitis, Crohn's disease, and multiple sclerosis.[24-26] As stated in Chapter 5, the presence of immune complexes is thought to contribute greatly to the disease process in rheumatoid arthritis. Experimental and clinical studies have shown that protease enzyme preparations are extremely effective in reducing circulating immune complex levels. Clinical improvements correspond with decreases in immune complex levels.

Most of the clinical studies using pancreatic enzyme preparations in the treatment of inflammatory or autoimmune diseases have utilized enzyme preparations that are weak in potency when compared to a number of enzyme preparations available in the United States. Table 6.1 offers a comparison of an enzyme preparation used in Germany—a preparation that has proven effective—and a popular U.S. enzyme version. Presumably, by using a higher-potency product, the impressive results demonstrated by weaker preparations can be improved upon.

Table 6.1 Comparison of Ingredients in Popular Pancreatic Enzyme Preparations

	Popular U.S. Version (mg)	German Version (mg)
Pancreatin*		
10X	325	
1X		100
Papain	50	60 mg.
Bromelain	50	45
Trypsin	75	24
Lipase	10	10
Amylase	10	10
Chymotrypsin	2	1
Lysozyme	10	
Rutin		50

Pancreatin refers to preparations of pancreatic enzymes isolated from fresh hog pancreas.

Dosage of Pancreatic Enzyme Products

The level of enzyme activity of a particular pancreatic enzyme product is the primary determinant of its dosage. The United States Pharmacopeia (USP) has set strict definitions for the levels of activity. A 1X pancreatic enzyme (pancreatin) product has in each milligram not less than 25 USP units of amylase activity, not less than 2.0 USP units of lipase activity, and not less than 25 USP units of protease activity. Pancreatin of higher potency is given a whole-number multiple indicating its strength. For example, a full-strength undiluted pancreatic extract that is 10 times stronger than the USP standard would be referred to as 10X USP.

Full-strength products are preferred to lower-potency pancreatin products because lower-potency products are often diluted with salt, lactose, or galactose to achieve desired strength (for example, 4X or 1X). The dosage recommendation I make for a 10X USP pancreatic enzyme product in the treatment of rheumatoid arthritis is 500 to 1,000 milligrams, three times a day, 10 to 20 minutes before meals.

Enzyme products are often enteric-coated—that is to say, they are often coated to prevent digestion in the stomach, so that the enzymes will be liberated in the small intestine. However, numerous studies have shown that non–enteric-coated enzyme preparations actually outperform enteric-coated products if they are given prior to a meal or on an empty stomach.

Dietary Fats

The role of dietary fats in the promotion of the inflammatory process in rheumatoid arthritis is becoming clear. Fatty acids are important mediators of inflammation because of their ability to form inflammatory compounds known as prostaglandins, thromboxanes, and leukotrienes. Manipulation of dietary oil intake can significantly increase or decrease inflammation, depending on the type of oil. To appreciate the role that dietary fats play in rheumatoid arthritis, it is essential to have a good understanding of dietary fats in general.

Typically, saturated fats are animal fats that are semi-solid to solid at room temperature. Vegetable fats are liquid at room temperature and are referred to as unsaturated fats or oils. Figure 6.4 presents an example of a saturated fat, stearic acid.

Stearic acid is an 18-carbon saturated fatty acid that is carrying as many carbon molecules as it can. Figure 6.5 shows oleic acid, an 18-carbon mono-unsaturated fatty acid. It is missing two hydrogen molecules, leaving two carbon molecules unsaturated. This causes the carbons to bind to each other to form a double bond.

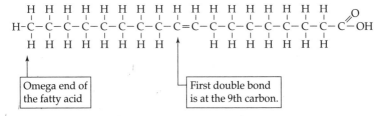

Figure 6.4 Stearic acid

Figure 6.5 Oleic acid, an omega-9 oil

Oleic acid is a mono-unsaturated fatty acid because it contains one double bond at the ninth carbon molecule. In a shorthand way, *oleic acid* is written $C_{18:1\omega9}$ or $C18:1\omega9$. This means that oleic acid is a carbon chain that contains 18 carbons and one double bond. Oleic acid is termed an omega-9 oil because its first unsaturated bond occurs at the ninth carbon from the omega end.

Linoleic acid is an 18-carbon polyunsaturated fatty acid. As Figure 6.6 shows, it contains more than one double bond; it has two. *Linoleic acid* would be written $C18:2\omega6$. Linoleic acid is classified as an omega-6 oil because the first double bond occurs at the sixth carbon.

Alpha-linolenic acid is an 18-carbon polyunsaturated fatty acid with three double bonds, $C18:3\omega3$. Alpha-linolenic acid, shown in Figure 6.7, is an omega-3 oil.

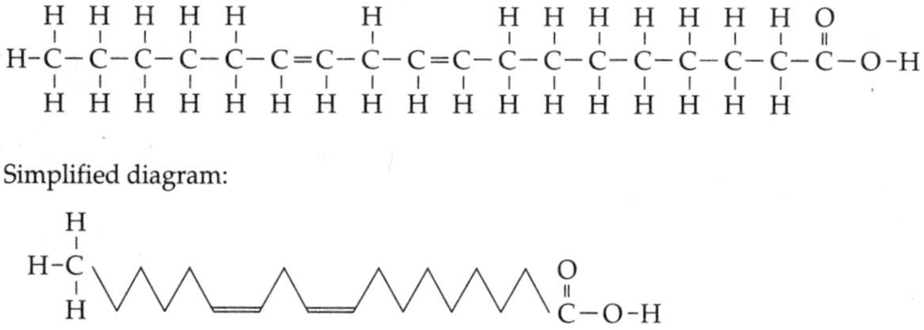

Simplified diagram:

Figure 6.6   Linoleic acid, an omega-6 oil

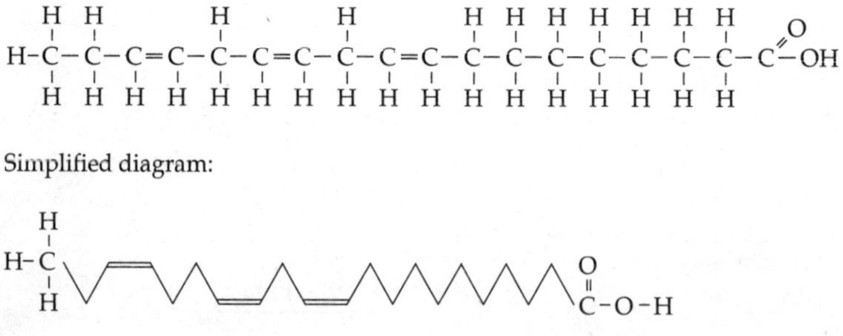

Simplified diagram:

Figure 6.7   Alpha-linolenic acid, an omega-3 oil

The balance of omega-6 to omega-3 oils is critical to proper prostaglandin metabolism. Prostaglandins and related compounds are hormonelike molecules derived from 20-carbon fatty acid chains that contain three, four, or five double bonds. Linoleic and linolenic acids can be converted to prostaglandins by the addition of two carbon molecules and the removal of hydrogen molecules (if necessary). Figure 6.8 shows the steps in prostaglandin metabolism. The number of double bonds in the fatty acid determines the classification of the prostaglandin.

Series 1 and 2 prostaglandins come from the omega-6 fatty acids, with the linoleic acid serving as the starting point. Linoleic acid is changed to gamma-linolenic acid and then dihomo-gamma-linolenic acid (DHGLA), which contains three double bonds and is the precursor to prostaglandins of the 1 series. Dihomo-gamma-linolenic acid can also be converted to arachidonic acid, which contains four double bonds and is precursor to the series 2 prostaglandins. However, because delta-5 desaturase, the enzyme responsible for the conversion of DHGLA to arachidonic acid, prefers the omega-3 oils, the greatest source of arachidonic acid for humans is the diet. Arachidonic acid is found almost entirely in animal foods, along with saturated fats.

Arachidonic acid contributes greatly to the inflammatory process through its conversion to inflammatory prostaglandins and leukotrienes. The reason vegetarian diets are often beneficial in the treatment of inflammatory conditions such as rheumatoid arthritis is presumably that the lack of meat decreases the availability of arachidonic acid for conversion to inflammatory prostaglandins and leukotrienes.[9,10]

Another important way of decreasing the inflammatory response is promotion of the omega-3 prostaglandin pathway. This pathway can begin with linolenic acid, an essential fatty acid that can be eventually converted to eicosapentaenoic acid, or EPA, which is the precursor to series 3 prostaglandins. This means that, although EPA is found

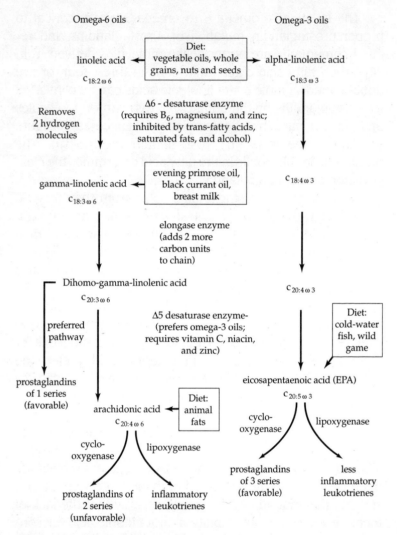

Figure 6.8 Prostaglandin metabolism

preformed in cold-water fish (such as salmon, mackerel, and herring), certain vegetable oils (flaxseed and canola, for example), by providing linolenic acid, can also increase body EPA and series 3 prostaglandin levels.

The net effect of consumption of omega-3 oils is a significantly reduced inflammatory or allergic response. Several clinical studies have demonstrated a therapeutic effect from supplementing the diet with EPA (1.8 grams daily) or cod liver oil.[2,3,27–29] However, supplementation may not be necessary if a serving of one of these cold-water fish is consumed at least once daily. For vegetarians, flaxseed oil may provide similar benefit to that of EPA, although the research behind this recommendation is not as solid.[30] Nonetheless, keep in mind that a vegetarian diet alone is therapeutic for many rheumatoid arthritis sufferers. Table 6.2 shows the fatty acid composition of selected foods and oils.

GLA Versus Omega-3 Oils

Black currant, borage, and evening primrose oils contain gamma-linolenic acid (GLA), an omega-6 oil. These oils are often recommended by nutritional-oriented physicians for the treatment of inflammatory conditions, such as rheumatoid arthritis and eczema. GLA is a precursor to series 1 DHGLA and prostaglandins. Unlike the pro-inflammatory series 2 prostaglandins, which are derived from arachidonic acid, series 1 prostaglandins exert anti-inflammatory effects. In addition, other derivatives of DHGLA actually block the formation of damaging leukotrienes.[2,3] These biochemical effects have provided the rationale behind supplementing the diet with black currant, borage, or evening primrose oil.

Several clinical trials have sought to determine the effectiveness of GLA supplementation on the course of rheumatoid arthritis.[2,3,31,32] Most of the studies have used evening primrose oil. The results of the studies have been conflicting. Some studies have shown some benefit; others have not. My belief is that, to be effective, GLA supplementation must accompany restriction of arachidonic acid intake and supplementation of omega-3 oils. However, even this recommendation may not produce beneficial effects. One study indicated that GLA supplementation can actually increase the level of arachidonic acid in the body while reducing the level of EPA.[33] Individuals may be better off using flaxseed oil.

Table 6.2   Fat Content and Fatty Acid Composition of Selected Foods and Vegetable Oils

Food	Fat Content (%)	Fatty Acid Composition (% of total fats)			
		Linolenic Acid	Linoleic Acid	Oleic Acid	Saturated Fats
Almond	54	0	17	78	5
Brazil nut	67	0	24	48	24
Canola	30	7	30	54	7
Cashew	42	0	6	70	18
Coconut	35	0	3	6	91
Corn	4	0	59	24	17
Filbert	62	0	16	54	5
Flaxseed	35	58	14	19	9
Macadamia nut	72	0	10	71	12
Olive	20	0	8	76	16
Peanut	48	0	29	47	18
Pecan	71	0	20	63	7
Pistachio	54	0	19	65	9
Pumpkin seed	47	15	42	34	9
Rice bran	10	0	35	48	17
Sesame seed	49	0	45	42	13
Soy	18	9	50	26	15
Sunflower	47	0	65	23	12
Walnut	60	5	51	28	16

Flaxseed Oil: The Best Choice

In my opinion, the best choice for an oil supplement in the treatment of rheumatoid arthritis is flaxseed oil—especially when cost is taken into consideration. The recommended daily dosage of either EPA (1.8 grams) or GLA supplements

(5 grams) costs $50 to $100 per month. Taking less than the recommended dosage is not likely to produce benefit. In contrast, flaxseed oil is fairly inexpensive. A 12-ounce bottle of flaxseed oil costs less than $12. At a daily dose of 1 tablespoon, this 12-ounce bottle would last more than a month. This daily dose of a high-quality flaxseed oil provides about 6 grams of alpha-linolenic acid and 2 grams of linoleic acid.

Homemade salad dressings are the perfect opportunity to use flaxseed oil. In *The Healing Power of Foods Cookbook* (Prima Publishing, Rocklin, CA, 1993), I give several recipes for salad dressings. In this book, see Chapter 7 for a recipe for Herb Dressing.

The Importance of Dietary Antioxidants

The importance of consuming a diet rich in fresh fruits and vegetables cannot be overstated in the dietary treatment of rheumatoid arthritis. These foods are the best sources of dietary antioxidants. As antioxidant nutrients, the benefits of vitamin C, beta-carotene, vitamin E, selenium, and zinc are becoming well recognized and well accepted. Still other plant compounds promote healthy joints, however. In short, the antioxidant benefits of fresh fruits and vegetables go well beyond the antioxidant effects of vitamins and minerals. Of particular benefit in the treatment of rheumatoid arthritis are flavonoids.

Flavonoids

The flavonoids are a group of plant pigments largely responsible for the colors of fruits and flowers. However, they serve more than aesthetic functions. In plants, flavonoids protect against environmental stress. In humans, flavonoids appear to function as biological response modifiers.

In other words, flavonoids appear to modify the body's reaction to compounds such as allergens, viruses, and carcinogens. Flavonoids have anti-inflammatory, anti-allergic, antiviral, and anticancer properties.[34-36] Flavonoid molecules are unique in that they are active against a wide variety of oxidants and free radicals.

Recent research suggests that flavonoids may be useful in the support of many health conditions. In fact, many of the medicinal actions of foods, juices, herbs, pollens, and propolis (a resinous material collected by bees from trees and buds) are now known to be directly related to their flavonoid content. Over 4,000 flavonoid compounds have been characterized and classified according to chemical structure.

Different foods provide different flavonoids and different benefits. For example, the flavonoids responsible for the colors of blueberries, blackberries, cherries, grapes, hawthorn berries, and many flowers are termed anthocyanidins and proanthocyanidins. These flavonoids are found in the flesh of the fruit as well as the skin, and they prompt very strong "vitamin P" activity.[37] Among these are the abilities to increase vitamin C levels within cells, decrease the leakiness and breakage of small blood vessels, protect against free radical damage, and support joint structures.

These flavonoids have a very beneficial effect on collagen. Collagen is the most abundant protein of the body and is responsible for maintaining the integrity of "ground substance." Ground substance is responsible for holding together the tissues of the body. Collagen is also found in tendons, ligaments, and cartilage. Collagen is destroyed during inflammatory processes that occur in rheumatoid arthritis, gout, and other inflammatory conditions involving bones, joints, cartilage, and other connective tissue. Anthocyanidins and other flavonoids affect collagen metabolism in many ways:

- They have the unique ability to actually cross-link collagen fibers, resulting in reinforcement of the natural cross-linking of collagen that forms the collagen matrix of connective tissue (ground substance, cartilage, tendon, and the like).
- They prevent free radical damage, because they scavenge antioxidants and free radicals.
- They inhibit enzymes secreted by white blood cells— enzymes that would otherwise destroy collagen structures during inflammation.
- They prevent the release and synthesis of compounds, such as histamine, that promote inflammation.

These remarkable effects on collagen structures and the potent antioxidant activity of berry flavonoids make them extremely important in the treatment of any form of arthritis. As mentioned in Chapter 4, cherries can be of great benefit in the treatment of gout.[38] If you have any form of arthritis, increase your consumption of cherries and other rich sources of flavonoids. It also may be wise to use flavonoid supplements. Flavonoids, such as quercetin, have anti-inflammatory effects, especially when combined with proteolytic enzymes.[39,40] Table 6.3 shows the flavonoid content of selected foods.

Supplements for the Treatment of Rheumatoid Arthritis

A number of individual nutrients have been shown to be of benefit to people with rheumatoid arthritis. Most of these nutrients are involved in key antioxidant systems, again highlighting the importance of a diet rich in plant foods. Here are brief descriptions of and recommendations regarding

Table 6.3 Flavonoid Content of Selected Foods (mg/3½-oz [100-g] serving)

Foods	4-Oxo-flavonoids*	Anthocyanins	Catechins[†]	Biflavans
Fruits				
Grapefruit	50			
Grapefruit juice	20			
Oranges, Valencia	50–100			
Orange juice	20–40			
Apples	3–16	1–2	20–75	50–90
Apple juice				15
Apricots	10–18		25	
Pears	1–5		5–20	1–3
Peaches		1–12	10–20	90–120
Tomatoes	85–130			
Blueberry		130–250	10–20	
Cherries, sour		45		25
Cherries, sweet			6–7	15
Cranberries	5	60–200	20	100
Cowberries		100	25	100–150
Currants, black	20–400	130–400	15	50
Currant juice		75–100		
Grapes, red		65–140	5–30	50
Plums, yellow		2–10		
Plums, blue		10–25	200	
Raspberries, black		300–400		
Raspberries, red		30–35		
Strawberries	20–100	15–35	30–40	
Hawthorn berries			200–800	
Vegetables				
Cabbage, red		25		
Onions	100–2,000	0–25		
Parsley	1,400			
Rhubarb		200		

Foods	4-Oxo-flavonoids*	Anthocyanins	Catechins†	Biflavans
Miscellaneous				
Beans, dry		10–1,000		
Sage	1,000–1,500			
Tea	5–50		10–500	100–200
Wine, red	2–4	50–120	100–150	·100–250

*4-oxo-flavonoids: the sum of flavanones, flavones, and flavanols (including quercetin)
†Catechins include proanthocyanins
SOURCE: Kuhnau J: The flavonoids: A class of semi-essential food components: Their role in human nutrition. World R Nutr and Diet 24:117–91, 1976.

nutrients that cause positive effects in the treatment of rheumatoid arthritis.

Selenium and Vitamin E

Patients with rheumatoid arthritis have low selenium levels.[41–43] Selenium plays an important role as an antioxidant and serves as the mineral cofactor in the free radical-scavenging enzyme glutathione peroxidase. This enzyme is especially important in reducing the production of inflammatory prostaglandins and leukotrienes. In addition, selenium has a synergistic effect with other antioxidant mechanisms.

Because free radicals, oxidants, prostaglandins, and leukotrienes cause much of the tissue damage associated with rheumatoid arthritis, a deficiency of selenium results in even more significant damage.

Clinical studies have not yet clearly demonstrated that selenium supplementation alone improves the signs and symptoms of rheumatoid arthritis. However, one clinical study indicated that selenium combined with vitamin E had a positive effect.[43] Vitamin E is an important antioxidant, working synergistically with selenium.

Because patients with rheumatoid arthritis have an increased demand for selenium and vitamin E, supplementing the daily diet with 50 to 200 micrograms of selenium and 200 to 400 international units (IU) of vitamin E appears to be appropriate. Most quality multiple-vitamin, multiple-mineral formulas provide the recommended amounts of vitamin E and selenium.

The selenium content of foods varies widely. The best sources are fish and grains. However, the amount of selenium in grains and other plant foods is directly related to the amount of selenium available in the soil.

Zinc

Zinc has antioxidant effects, and it functions in the antioxidant enzyme copper-zinc superoxide dismutase (copper-zinc SOD). Zinc levels are typically reduced in patients with rheumatoid arthritis. Several studies have used zinc in the treatment of rheumatoid arthritis; some have demonstrated a slight therapeutic effect.[44-46] Most of the studies utilized zinc in the form of sulfate. Better results may be produced by using a form of zinc with a higher absorption rate, such as zinc picolinate, zinc monomethionine, or zinc citrate. In addition to eating foods rich in zinc—foods such as whole grains, nuts, and seeds—individuals with rheumatoid arthritis should supplement their diet with an additional 30 to 45 milligrams of zinc daily—preferably, one of the more absorbable forms of zinc. Most quality multiple-vitamin, multiple-mineral formulas provide this amount of zinc.

Manganese and Superoxide Dismutase

You have already read about the antioxidant enzyme copper-zinc superoxide dismutase (copper-zinc SOD). Manganese functions in a different form of SOD, manganese SOD.

Patients with rheumatoid arthritis are deficient in manganese SOD.[47] The injectable form of this enzyme (available in Europe) has been shown to be effective in the treatment of rheumatoid arthritis.[48] However, it is not clear if any orally administered SOD can escape digestion in the intestinal tract and exert a therapeutic effect. In one study, oral SOD had no effect on tissue SOD levels.[49]

Perhaps a better and more economical method of raising SOD is simply to supplement the diet with additional manganese. Manganese supplementation has been shown to increase SOD activity, indicating increased antioxidant activity.[50] Although no clinical studies have been conducted to determine the effectiveness of manganese supplementation in the treatment of rheumatoid arthritis, supplementation seems indicated because patients with rheumatoid arthritis have low levels of manganese. The standard recommendation for patients with rheumatoid arthritis is daily supplementation with 5 to 15 milligrams of manganese. Dietary sources of manganese include nuts, whole grains, dried fruits, and green leafy vegetables. Meats, dairy products, poultry, and seafood are poor sources of manganese.

Vitamin C

Vitamin C functions as an important antioxidant. Concentrations of vitamin C in white blood cells and plasma are significantly decreased in rheumatoid arthritis patients.[51] Supplementation with vitamin C increases SOD activity, decreases histamine levels, and provides some anti-inflammatory action.[52,53] In addition to consuming foods rich in vitamin C—foods such as broccoli, Brussels sprouts, cabbage, citrus fruits, tomatoes, and berries—patients with rheumatoid arthritis should supplement the diet with an additional 1,000 to 3,000 milligrams of vitamin C daily, in divided dosages.

Pantothenic Acid

Compared to normal controls, the level of pantothenic acid in whole blood is low in patients with rheumatoid arthritis. In addition, disease activity is inversely correlated with pantothenic acid levels: The lower the level of pantothenic acid, the more severe the arthritis symptoms. Correction of low pantothenic acid levels brings about some alleviation of symptoms.[54]

In one double-blind study, subjective improvement was noted in patients receiving 2 grams of calcium pantothenate daily. Patients noted improvements in duration of morning stiffness, degree of disability, and severity of pain.[55] Dietary sources of pantothenic acid are whole grains and legumes. But, to reach the daily dose of 2 grams used in the clinical study, supplementation is required.

Iron

Anemia is quite common in patients with rheumatoid arthritis. Most common iron supplements, however, may actually do more harm than good. There are two forms of dietary iron, heme iron and nonheme iron. Heme iron may be useful to some patients with rheumatoid arthritis. Nonheme iron may actually increase inflammation.[56]

Heme iron is iron bound to hemoglobin and myoglobin. Nonheme iron includes the iron found in plant foods and iron salts such as ferrous fumarate, ferrous gluconate, and ferrous sulfate. Dietary sources of heme iron are animal meats, egg yolks, fish, and shellfish. Liver is regarded as the best dietary source of heme iron.

Heme iron is the most efficiently absorbed form of iron. About 25% of heme iron can be absorbed. Nonheme iron is poorly absorbed; its approximate absorption rate is 5%.[57] However, it is not the relatively high absorption rate of heme iron that makes it beneficial to individuals with rheumatoid arthritis. Heme iron is comparatively beneficial because un-bound iron (nonheme iron) can actually generate free radicals and pro-oxidants. Also, in most chronic diseases involving anemia, the anemia is simply unresponsive to nonheme iron. In contrast, heme iron supplementation is usually quite effec-tive in treating anemia, as it is in treating the anemia that may accompany rheumatoid arthritis.

The best iron supplement rheumatoid arthritis patients with iron-deficiency anemia can use is one made from liver extracts. In my opinion, the best liver product available is Liquid Liver Extract from Enzymatic Therapy. This extract is produced from a specific fraction of beef liver obtained from animals raised in South America, where ranchers use no chemical sprays, pesticides, or antibiotics in their livestock feed. The fats and cholesterol of the liver are removed via a special cold process, and then the extract is placed into gelatin capsules in free form (this ensures optimum utiliza-tion by the body). Liquid Liver Extract is far superior to liver and desiccated liver tablets.

Thymus Extracts

The thymus is the major gland of the human immune system. It is composed of two soft pinkish gray lobes lying in a bib-like fashion just below the thyroid gland and above the heart. To a very large extent, the health of the thymus determines the health of the immune system. Individuals with rheuma-toid arthritis have altered thymus gland and immune system function.

In the treatment of rheumatoid arthritis, it is necessary to employ measures designed to improve thymus function. Pro-moting optimal thymus gland activity can involve (1) in-creasing the dietary intake of antioxidant nutrients such as carotenes, vitamin C, vitamin E, zinc, and selenium; (2) sup-plementing the diet with nutrients required in the manufac-ture or action of thymic hormones (zinc, vitamin B6, and vitamin C); and (3) using products containing concentrates of calf thymus tissue. Of calf-tissue concentrates, bovine concentrates are the most common. (The term *calf,* in this context, can refer to the young of several different animals.)

Clinical trials have shown that oral administration of calf thymus concentrates, which are rich in thymus-derived polypeptides, are effective in (1) preventing recurrent respiratory infections in children; (2) correcting the T-cell defects in human immunodeficiency virus (AIDS) infections; (3) treating acute hepatitis B infections; (4) restoring the number of peripheral leukocytes in cancer patients whose white blood cell counts have been reduced by chemotherapy; and (5) treating allergies, including asthma, hay fever, and food allergies in children.[58,59]

The effectiveness of an orally administered thymus concentrate used for the listed conditions is due to broad immune system enhancement that, presumably, improved thymus function mediates. It is well established that the thymus produces a number of hormones that regulate the production and function of the immune system. Thymus gland dysfunction is thought to be responsible for the immune system derangement seen in many diseases.

The positive effect of orally administered thymus extracts supports the basic concept of glandular therapy: that the oral ingestion of glandular material of a certain animal gland will strengthen the corresponding human gland. The result is a broad general effect indicative of improved glandular function. It is interesting that thymus extract has been shown to normalize the ratio of T-helper cells to suppressor cells, regardless of the cause of the abnormal ratio. The ratio may be low (as in AIDS, chronic infections, and cancer) or high (as in rheumatoid arthritis, allergies, and migraine headaches).[58,59]

In the case of rheumatoid arthritis, a high T-helper cell to suppressor cell ratio results in increased antibody formation in joint tissues. The higher the ratio, the higher the number of antibodies being produced to damage joint structures. In one clinical study, rheumatoid arthritis patients with a helper to suppressor ratio of 3.3 achieved normal ratios (1.02 to 2.46) after three months of therapy with a thymus extract.[58]

The dosage of thymus extract varies from one manufacturer to another. The daily dose should be equivalent to 120 milligrams of pure polypeptides, with molecular weights less than 10,000 milligrams, or roughly 500 milligrams, of the crude polypeptide fraction. From a practical view, products concentrated and standardized for polypeptide content are preferable to crude freeze-dried preparations.

Although use of a thymus extract may not result in clinical improvement, it appears to be useful in restoring proper immune function.

Plant-Based Medicines for Rheumatoid Arthritis

Many plants possess significant anti-inflammatory action and are appropriate in the treatment of rheumatoid arthritis. The plants discussed in this section are some of the more effective. Also discussed are plants that can enhance the function or secretion of the body's own cortisone and those that can prevent or reverse some of the negative effects of orally administered cortisone. The herbal medicines are presented in order according to my ranking of their importance in treating rheumatoid arthritis.

Curcumin

Curcumin, the yellow pigment of turmeric (*Curcuma longa*), appears to be one of nature's most potent anti-inflammatory agents. Turmeric is the major ingredient of curry powder and is also used in prepared mustard. It is used extensively in foods for both its color and flavor. In addition, turmeric is used in the Chinese and Indian (Ayurvedic) systems of medicine as an anti-inflammatory agent.

Turmeric and its derivatives can produce a great deal of pharmacological activity.[60] Curcumin is a powerful antioxidant, and its ability to prevent free radical damage is greater than that of vitamin C, vitamin E, or SOD.[61-63] However, the protection curcumin provides against inflammation and joint damage is only partially explained by its direct antioxidant effect and scavenging of free radicals. Additional effects include enhancement of the body's natural antioxidant system and the body's anti-inflammatory mechanisms.

Numerous studies have demonstrated the exceptional anti-inflammatory effects of curcumin.[60,63-65] In models of acute inflammation, curcumin is as effective as cortisone or the potent anti-inflammatory drug phenylbutazone.[63-65] However, phenylbutazone and cortisone are associated with significant toxicity; curcumin is without side effects.

Among the many direct anti-inflammatory effects of curcumin is the formation of leukotrienes and other mediators of inflammation.[66-68] As for its indirect effects, models of chronic inflammation show that curcumin is much less active in animals that have had their adrenal glands removed. This means that curcumin works to enhance the body's anti-inflammatory mechanisms. Possible mechanisms of action include (1) stimulating the release of adrenal corticosteroids; (2) "sensitizing," or priming, cortisone receptor sites, thereby facilitating cortisone action; and (3) preventing cortisone breakdown.

In comparisons with standard drugs, curcumin has demonstrated some beneficial effects in human studies. In one double-blind clinical trial involving patients with rheumatoid arthritis, the effects of curcumin (1,200 milligrams per day) were compared to those of phenylbutazone (300 milligrams per day).[69] The improvements in the duration of morning stiffness, walking time, and joint swelling were comparable in both groups. However, phenylbutazone is associated with significant adverse effects; at the recommended dosage curcumin has not been shown to produce any side effects.

Another study used a new human model, the postoperative inflammation model, for evaluating NSAIDs. Again, curcumin exerted anti-inflammatory action comparable to that of phenylbutazone.[70]

Note that, though curcumin has an anti-inflammatory effect similar to that of phenylbutazone and various NSAIDs, it does not possess direct analgesic action.

The studies cited indicate that curcumin can provide benefit in the treatment of the flare-ups of inflammation caused by rheumatoid arthritis. Furthermore, compared to standard drug treatment, curcumin is safer and better tolerated. No toxicity reactions to curcumin have been reported. Animals fed very high levels of curcumin (3 grams per kilogram of body weight) have not exhibited any significant adverse effects.[71]

The recommended dosage of curcumin as an anti-inflammatory is 400 to 600 milligrams, three times a day. To achieve a similar amount of curcumin using turmeric would require a dosage of 8,000 to 60,000 milligrams. Because the absorption of orally administered curcumin is in question, curcumin is often formulated in conjunction with bromelain to possibly enhance absorption. In addition, bromelain has anti-inflammatory effects of its own (see the next section). If you use a curcumin-bromelain combination, take it on an empty stomach, 20 minutes before meals or between meals.

Providing curcumin in a lipid base—such as lecithin, fish oils, or essential fatty acids—may also increase absorption. If you use this form, take it with meals.

Bromelain

Bromelain refers to a mixture of enzymes found in pineapple. Bromelain was introduced as a medicinal agent in 1957, and since that time over two hundred scientific papers about its therapeutic applications have appeared in medical literature.[72] These studies report that bromelain exerts a wide variety of beneficial effects, including reduction of inflammation in cases of rheumatoid arthritis.[73] Figure 6.9 lists the conditions that bromelain can be effective in treating.

Several mechanisms may account for bromelain's anti-inflammatory effects, including the inhibition of pro-inflammatory compounds. Bromelain can prevent swelling by activating compounds that break down fibrin. (Fibrin was discussed early in this chapter, in the section about the importance of proteases.) Also, bromelain blocks the production of kinins. Kinins are compounds produced during inflammation. They increase swelling as well as cause pain.

Angina

Arthritis

Athletic injury

Bronchitis

Bruises

Burn debridement

Maldigestion

Menstrual cramps

Pancreatic insufficiency

Pneumonia

Rheumatoid arthritis

Scleroderma

Sinusitis

Surgical trauma

Thrombophlebitis

Figure 6.9   Conditions in which bromelain has documented clinical efficacy

The standard dosage of bromelain is based on its mcu (milk clotting unit) activity. The most beneficial range of activity appears to be 1,800 to 2,000 mcu. The dosage that can effect this level is 400 to 600 milligrams, three times daily, on an empty stomach. Although most studies have utilized commercially prepared bromelain, it is conceivable that drinking fresh pineapple juice could exert similar, if not superior, benefits. One of the best fresh juices to consume if you have rheumatoid arthritis is pineapple-ginger. Simply juice one-half of a pineapple along with a ¼-inch slice of fresh ginger. For additional fresh juice recommendations for rheumatoid arthritis, consult *The Complete Book of Juicing* (Michael T. Murray, Prima Publishing, Rocklin, CA, 1992).

Ginger

Although ginger (*Zingiber officinale*) is native to southern Asia, it is now extensively cultivated in the tropics (for example, India, China, Jamaica, Haiti, and Nigeria). Jamaica is a major exporter of the crop. Jamaica exports ginger to all parts of the world—more than 2 million pounds annually.

The knotted and branched underground stem, or rhizome (commonly called the root), is the portion of ginger used for culinary and medicinal purposes. Ginger has been used as a medicine for thousands of years in China. Chinese records dating from the fourth century B.C. indicate that it was used to treat numerous conditions, including rheumatism.

Ginger causes numerous pharmacological activities. The most relevant in terms of rheumatoid arthritis are its antioxidant effects; its ability to inhibit synthesis of prostaglandin, thromboxane, and leukotrienes; and its anti-inflammatory effects. In the treatment of rheumatoid arthritis, fresh ginger may be more effective in treating inflammation than dried preparations, because fresh ginger contains a protease that may cause actions similar to those of bromelain.[74-76]

A preliminary clinical study involved seven patients with rheumatoid arthritis. For all seven, conventional drugs had provided only temporary or partial relief.[77] All patients were treated with ginger. One patient took 50 grams per day of lightly cooked ginger; the remaining six took either 5 grams of fresh or 0.1 to 1 gram of powdered ginger daily. Despite the difference in dosage, all patients reported substantial improvement, including pain relief, joint mobility, and decrease in swelling and morning stiffness.

A follow-up study evaluated 28 patients with rheumatoid arthritis, 18 with osteoarthritis, and 10 with muscular discomfort. All had been taking powdered ginger for periods ranging from 3 months to 2½ years.[78] Based on clinical observations, 75% of the arthritis patients and 100% of the patients with muscular discomfort experienced relief from pain or swelling. The recommended dosage was 500 to 1,000 milligrams per day, but many patients took three to four times that amount. Patients taking the higher dosages reported quicker relief and better results.

Many questions remain concerning the best form of ginger and the proper dosage. Most scientific studies have utilized 1 gram of dry powdered ginger root. This amount is a relatively small dose of ginger compared to the average daily dose of 8 to 10 grams consumed in India.

Although most scientific studies have used powdered ginger root, fresh (or possibly freeze-dried) ginger root at an equivalent dosage may yield even better results because it contains higher levels of gingerol as well as the active protease.

In light of all this information, what is a practical dosage of ginger for those with rheumatoid arthritis? A daily dosage of 2 to 4 grams of dry powdered ginger may be effective. This amount would be equivalent to approximately 20 grams, or ⅔ ounce, of fresh ginger root—that's roughly a ½-inch slice. These amounts of ginger can easily be incorporated into the diet, especially if you have a juicer. At this dosage, ginger does not appear to have any side effects.

Chinese Thoroughwax

The root of Chinese thoroughwax (*Bupleurum falcatum*) is an important component in various traditional Chinese medicines, particularly remedies for inflammatory conditions. Recently these formulas have been used in combination with corticosteroid drugs such as prednisone.[79] Chinese thoroughwax has been shown to enhance the activity of cortisone.

The active constituents of Chinese thoroughwax are steroidlike compounds known as saikosaponins. These compounds cause diverse pharmacological activity, including significant anti-inflammatory action.[79,80] The saikosaponins apparently increase the release of cortisone and other hormones by the adrenal gland and potentiate their effects. Saikosaponins have also been shown to prevent adrenal gland atrophy caused by corticosteroid drugs.[81] Some studies have recommended that patients on corticosteroid drugs take herbal formulas containing Chinese thoroughwax, to help protect the adrenal gland.[79]

The root of licorice(*Glycyrrhiza glabra*) and *Panax ginseng* appear to enhance the action of Chinese thoroughwax, and the three are almost always used together in traditional Chinese herbal formulas. Both licorice root and ginseng have components with anti-inflammatory activity.[82] In addition, these herbs have been shown to improve the health of the adrenal glands.

Perhaps the major effect of licorice is its ability to inhibit the breakdown of adrenal hormones by the liver. When used in combination with Chinese thoroughwax, the net effect is increased corticosteroids: The Chinese thoroughwax promotes secretion of these hormones by the adrenal glands, and the licorice root slows their destruction by the liver.

If you are currently taking corticosteroids or have taken them in the past, take a plant-based formula that supplies adrenal restoratives. For example, in my clinical practice I prescribe capsules that contain extracts of the following:

	Mg
Chinese thoroughwax (*Bupleurum falcatum*)	150
Licorice root (4:1) (*Glycyrrhiza glabra*)	50
Curcuma root* (*Curcuma longa*)	50
Korean ginseng root (*Panax ginseng*)	100
Siberian ginseng root† (*Eleutherococcus senticosus*)	100
Mexican yam extract (10:1) (*Dioscorea spinosa*)	100

*Standardized to contain 2.5% curcumin
†Standardized to contain more than 1% eleutheroside E

The dosage of this formula is 2 capsules, three times daily, when a person is on corticosteroids. If a person needs to rebuild the adrenals, he or she should take this formula for a minimum of three months.

Boswellia

Boswellia serrata was discussed in Chapter 2, as a natural approach to osteoarthritis. According to unpublished clinical trials, boswellic acid extracts have caused positive results in rheumatoid arthritis. In one study, 175 patients with rheumatoid arthritis were treated with a boswellic acid extract for four weeks. Of those patients, 14% exhibited excellent results; 44%, good results; and 30%, fair results. Only 3% exhibited poor results.[83] The standard dosage for boswellic acids in arthritis is 400 milligrams, three times daily. No side effects due to boswellic acids have been reported.

Feverfew

Because feverfew (*Chrysanthemum parthenium*) has a long folk history in the treatment of fever, arthritis, and migraine, it's only natural to assume that this herb acts in a fashion similar to that of aspirin. Indeed, in experimental models of inflammation, researchers have actually shown that extracts of feverfew are more effective at inhibiting inflammation and fever than aspirin.[84,85] Feverfew extracts inhibit the synthesis of many pro-inflammatory compounds at the initial stage of synthesis. Feverfew also decreases the secretion of inflammatory chemicals from platelets and white blood cells. The net effect of feverfew's action is a significantly decreased inflammatory response.

Although a double-blind, placebo-controlled study demonstrated no apparent benefit from oral feverfew in the treatment of rheumatoid arthritis, the dosage used was extremely small (76 milligrams of dried, powdered feverfew leaf—about two medium-sized leaves) and patients continued to take NSAIDs, a practice that most likely reduced the efficacy of the feverfew.[86]

Scientists know that, in the treatment of migraine headaches, the effectiveness of feverfew depends on adequate levels of parthenolide, the active ingredient.[87,88] The preparations used in the clinical trials where feverfew exhibited a therapeutic effect had a parthenolide content of 0.2%. Recent chemical analysis of commercially available sources indicated that the parthenolide content of many popular products is insufficient to produce desirable results.[89] For this reason, consumers should look for feverfew products that state the level of parthenolide.

The migraine studies used low dosages of feverfew (50 milligrams per day). Higher dosages are probably necessary in the treatment of rheumatoid arthritis. Recommended dosages for rheumatoid arthritis patients follow.

Dosage (take these amounts, three times daily)

Dried leaves or by infusion (tea)	1 to 2 grams
Fluid extract (1:1)	1.0 to 2.0 milliliters (¼ to ½ teaspoon)
Freeze-dried leaf with a parthenolide content	100 to 250 0.2% milligrams

Feverfew is extremely well tolerated and no serious side effects have ever been reported. However, chewing the leaves can result in small ulcerations in the mouth and swelling of the lips and tongue. This condition occurs in about 10% of users.

Yucca

A double-blind clinical trial in patients with rheumatoid arthritis indicated that an extract of yucca (*Yucca aborescens*) can exert a positive therapeutic effect.[90] Results were of gradual onset, and no direct anti-inflammatory effects of the yucca extract were noted. The research suggested that the results were due to indirect effects on gastrointestinal flora. This suggestion is interesting, since bacterial endotoxins have been shown to promote tissue destruction. It is entirely possible that yucca decreases bacterial endotoxin absorption and thus reduces inflammation. If this is the mechanism of action, other plants containing compounds similar to those in yucca—plants such as sarsaparilla root (*Smilax sarsaparilla*)—may produce similar benefit.

Dosage (take these amounts, three times daily)

Powdered yucca leaf	2 to 4 grams, or as a cup of tea
Fluid extract (1:1)	1 to 2 milliliters (¼ to ½ teaspoon)
Solid extract (4:1)	250 to 500 milligrams

Physical Therapy

Physical therapy has a major role in the management of patients with rheumatoid arthritis. Though not curative, proper physical management can improve patient comfort and preserve joint and muscle function. Heat is typically used to help relieve stiffness and pain, relax muscles, and increase range of motion. Moist heat (for example, moist packs, hot baths) is more effective than dry heat (such as that from a heating pad). Paraffin baths can be used if skin irritation from regular water immersion develops. Cold packs are of value during acute flare-ups.

Strengthening and range-of-motion exercises are important for improving and maintaining joint function, as well as for general health. Patients with well-developed disease and significant inflammation should begin with progressive, passive range-of-motion and isometric exercises. As inflammation is ameliorated, active range-of-motion and isotonic exercises are more appropriate.

Final Comments

Rheumatoid arthritis is an aggressive disease that needs aggressive treatment. Here is a hierarchy of the key natural measures to employ. In addition to rheumatoid arthritis, these same measures apply to other autoimmune diseases that can lead to arthritis—diseases such as ankylosing spondylitis, systemic lupus, and scleroderma.

1. The first step is therapeutic fasting or an elimination diet followed by careful reintroduction of foods. Note any symptom-producing foods and avoid them in the future.

2. Eliminate all animal products from the diet, with the exception of cold-water fish. Follow the dietary recommendations given in this chapter as well as the guidelines presented in Chapter 7.

3. Drink 16 to 24 ounces of fresh fruit and vegetable juice each day. This will provide a large intake of antioxidants. Grind and consume a ¼- to ½-inch slice of fresh ginger in the juice each day.

4. Take 1 to 2 tablespoons of flaxseed oil each day.

5. Determine if you need hydrochloric acid supplementation.

6. Take a 10X USP pancreatic enzyme product at a dosage of 500 to 1,000 milligrams, three times a day, 10 to 20 minutes before meals.

7. Take a high-potency multiple-vitamin, multiple-mineral supplement that provides the recommended levels of vitamin E, selenium, zinc, and manganese. Also take an additional 1,000 to 3,000 milligrams of vitamin C daily, in divided dosages.

8. On a regular basis use the physical therapy treatments discussed in this chapter.

9. Take a high-quality thymus preparation at the appropriate dosage.

10. Take a curcumin-bromelain formula at a dosage of 400 to 600 milligrams, three times daily, between meals.

11. If you are taking corticosteroids or have taken them for more than three months in the past, take a formula containing herbs that support the adrenal glands.

12. If additional support is required, take boswellic acids, feverfew, or yucca.

The severity of rheumatoid arthritis varies from one person to the next. In mild to moderate rheumatoid arthritis, the 12 measures listed previously are extremely effective on their own. In severe cases, NSAIDs and other drugs may be necessary. However, do not abandon the natural measures; they will enhance the effectiveness of the drugs, meaning you can use lower dosages of the drugs. When the use of drugs is necessary, be sure to use DGL (see Chapter 2) to prevent or protect against peptic ulcers.

If you follow the recommendations in this book and do not experience benefit, I urge you to consult a naturopathic physician (N.D.) or holistic medical doctor. To find a physician in your area, call or write:

The American Association of Naturopathic Physicians
P.O. Box 20386
Seattle, WA 98102
(206) 323-7610

or

The American Holistic Medical Association
4101 Lake Boone Trail, #201
Raleigh, NC 26707
(919) 787-5146

My final recommendation is to beware of natural "miracle" cures for rheumatoid arthritis. If a company is claiming to have a product that is effective, ask for references to the medical literature. Take this information to your doctor and discuss with him or her the appropriateness of the treatment in your case.

Dietary Guidelines

7

The Design of
a Healthful Diet

There is little debate that a healthful diet must be rich in whole "natural" and unprocessed foods. Of particular importance are plant foods, such as fruits, vegetables, grains, beans, seeds, and nuts. These foods contain not only valuable nutrients, but also dietary fiber and other compounds that have health-promoting properties. A diet rich in plant foods offers significant protection against the development of chronic degenerative problems, such as heart disease, cancer, diabetes, stroke, and arthritis.[1-3] Figure 7.1 lists diseases associated with a diet low in plant foods.

A Healthful Diet

Most people give very little thought to the design of their diet. They are motivated to eat by sensual needs rather than what their body requires. Health is largely a conscious decision. Awareness of what to eat, in what quantities, and healthful ways to prepare food is critical.

Metabolic: Obesity, diabetes, kidney stones, gallstones, gout

Cardiovascular: Hypertension, heart disease, stroke, varicose veins, deep vein thrombosis, pulmonary embolism

Gastrointestinal: Constipation, appendicitis, diverticulitis, diverticulosis, hemorrhoids, colon cancer, irritable bowel syndrome, ulcerative colitis, Crohn's disease

Other: Dental caries, autoimmune disorders (including multiple sclerosis), thyrotoxicosis, many skin conditions

---

Figure 7.1   Diseases associated with a diet low in plant foods

The American Dietetic Association, in conjunction with the American Diabetes Association and other groups, has developed the Exchange System, a convenient tool for the rapid estimation of the calorie, protein, fat, and carbohydrate content of a diet. Originally intended for use in designing dietary recommendations for diabetics, the Exchange System is now used to design virtually all therapeutic diets. The Exchange System does not place enough stress on the quality of food choices, however.

This chapter will present a system of diet design called the Healthy Exchange System. It is a more beneficial system than the Exchange System because it focuses on unprocessed, whole foods. The Healthy Exchange System is based on seven lists:

List 1	Vegetables
List 2	Fruits
List 3	Breads, cereals, and starchy vegetables
List 4	Legumes
List 5	Fats and oils
List 6	Milk
List 7	Meats, fish, cheese, and eggs

Lists 6 and 7—the milk and meat lists—are optional. All food portions within each list provide approximately the same calories, proteins, fats, and carbohydrates. (The fact that the servings are equal in this sense gives rise to the term *exchange*—for the most part, any item in one list can be exchanged for any item in the same list.)

To use the Healthy Exchange System, you begin by determining your body frame size. Knowing this allows you to calculate the number of calories you need each day to maintain yourself heathfully. Then you turn to the diets of the Healthy Exchange System. These are "menus" that tell you how many servings from each Healthy Exchange List you should eat to consume the number of calories appropriate for you. You must then decide whether you will be a vegan (someone who does not consume meat or dairy products) or an omnivore (someone who eats animal and vegetable substances). At each specific calorie level, the Healthy Exchange System offers a vegan and an omnivore diet. Later in this chapter, you will determine your frame size, calculate the number of daily calories you need, and examine each Exchange List in detail.

Because all food portions within each Exchange List provide approximately the same calories, proteins, fats, and carbohydrates per serving, it is easy to construct a diet that has the following components:

Carbohydrates	65% to 75% of total calories
Fats	15% to 25% of total calories
Protein	10% to 15% of total calories
Dietary fiber	At least 50 grams

Of the carbohydrates ingested, 90% should be complex carbohydrates or naturally occurring sugars. Limit intake of refined carbohydrates and concentrated sugars (including

Table 7.1   Macronutrient Composition Per Serving

Healthy Exchange System List	Protein (g)	Fat (g)	Carbohydrates (g)	Fiber (g)	Calories (kcal)
Vegetables	3.0	0.0	11.0	1.0–3.0	50
Fruits	0.0	0.0	20.0	1.0–3.0	80
Breads, etc.	2.0	0.0	15.0	1.0–4.0	70
Legumes	7.0	0.5	15.0	6.0–7.0	90
Fats and oils	0.0	5.0	0.0	0.0	45
Milk	8.0	0.0	12.0	0.0	80
Meats, etc.	7.0	3.0	0.0	0.0	55

honey, pasteurized fruit juices, and dried fruit, as well as sugar and white flour) to less than 10% of the total calorie intake. Table 7.1 shows the protein, fat, carbohydrate, and fiber composition per serving for each Exchange List.

How Many Calories Do You Need?

The first step in determining your caloric needs is to determine the size of your body frame. The next step is to determine ideal body weight and calculate the number of calories necessary to sustain that weight.

Determining Frame Size   Extend your arm and bend the forearm upward at a 90-degree angle. Keep the fingers straight and turn the inside of your wrist away from your body. Place the thumb and index finger of your other hand on the two prominent bones on either side of your elbow. Measure the space between your fingers with a tape measure. Table 7.2 presents data for men and women; choose the data appropriate for you. Find your height in the left column. Compare the measurement of the breadth of your elbow with

Table 7.2 Data for the Calculation of Body Frame Size

Height in 1" Heels	Elbow Breadth
Men	
5'2"–5'3"	2½–2⅞"
5'4"–5'7"	2⅝–2⅞"
5'8"–5'11"	2¾–3"
6'0"–6'3"	2¾–3⅛"
6'4"	2⅞–3¼"
Women	
4'10"–5'3"	2¼–2½"
5'4"–5'11"	2⅜–2⅝"
6'0"	2½–2¾"

the elbow measurement beside your height. The elbow measurements in the table are for medium-framed individuals. If the breadth of your elbow is smaller than the range cited in the table, you have a small frame; if it is larger, you have a large frame.

Now that you know the size of your body frame, you can determine the body weight appropriate for it.

Determining Ideal Body Weight   The most popular tables of "desirable" weight are those provided by the Metropolitan Life Insurance Company. The most recent edition of these tables, published in 1983, gives weight ranges for men and women, in 1-inch increments of height, for three body frame sizes. Table 7.3 presents the Metropolitan Life Insurance tables of desirable weight.

The next step in determining your daily caloric needs is to make a calculation involving weight and activity level.

Factoring In Your Activity Level   Convert your ideal weight in pounds to kilograms by multiplying it by 0.4536.

Table 7.3 1983 Metropolitan Life Insurance Tables of Ideal
Body Weight*

Height	Weight (lb)		
	Small Frame	Medium Frame	Large Frame
Men			
5'2"	128–134	131–141	138–150
5'3"	130–136	133–143	140–153
5'4"	132–138	135–145	142–156
5'5"	134–140	137–148	144–160
5'6"	136–142	139–151	146–164
5'7"	138–145	142–154	149–168
5'8"	140–148	145–157	152–172
5'9"	142–151	148–160	155–176
5'10"	144–154	151–163	158–180
5'11"	146–157	154–166	161–184
6'0"	149–160	157–170	164–188
6'1"	152–164	160–174	168–192
6'2"	155–168	164–178	172–197
6'3"	158–172	167–182	176–202
6'4"	162–176	171–187	181–207
Women			
4'10"	102–111	109–121	118–131
4'11"	103–113	111–123	120–134
5'0"	104–115	113–126	122–137
5'1"	106–118	115–129	125–140
5'2"	108–121	118–132	128–143
5'3"	111–124	121–135	131–147
5'4"	114–127	124–138	134–151
5'5"	117–130	127–141	137–155
5'6"	120–133	130–144	140–159
5'7"	123–136	133–147	143–163
5'8"	126–139	136–150	146–167
5'9"	129–142	139–153	149–170
5'10"	132–145	142–156	152–173
5'11"	135–148	145–159	155–176
6'0"	138–151	148–162	158–179

*Weights cited are, in pounds, for adults age 25–59, based on lowest mortality. Weight is cited according to frame size in indoor clothing (5 pounds for men and 3 pounds for women), wearing shoes with 1" heels.

Next choose, from the list that follows, the activity level that best describes you.

Little physical activity	30 calories
Light physical activity	35 calories
Moderate physical activity	40 calories
Heavy physical activity	45 calories

Make a note of the number of calories cited for the level you chose. You will use this number in the equation that calculates the number of calories you need each day. The equation follows.

Weight (in kg)	×	Number of calories for activity level	=	Approximate daily calorie requirements
____	×	____	=	____ calories

For example, I weigh 195 pounds. That amount multiplied by 0.4536 equals 88.452, or about 88 kilograms. I would rate my physical activity level as moderate. (Even though I exercise at least 5 days a week for a minimum of 1 hour, during most of the day I am sedentary.) Therefore, the equation to calculate my daily caloric needs looks like this:

$88 \times 40 = 3{,}520$ calories

Now that you know your daily caloric needs, you are ready to take a look at the diets of the Healthy Exchange System.

The Diets of the Healthy Exchange System

As you recall, the Healthy Exchange System defines seven lists—five mandatory and two optional—that categorize foods according to broad groups. The diets of the Healthy Exchange System define the number of servings you should eat from each list. The diets provide total daily calories in the range of 1,000 to 3,000 calories, in increments of 500 calories. The system offers two diets at each level: one for the vegan and one for the omnivore.

As an example of one of the diets, study the 1,500-calorie vegan diet, which follows.

1,500-Calorie Vegan Diet (daily intake)

List 1 (vegetables)	5 servings
List 2 (fruits)	2 servings
List 3 (breads, cereals, and starchy vegetables)	9 servings
List 4 (legumes)	2.5 servings
List 5 (fats and oils)	4 servings

This diet results in an intake of approximately 1,500 calories, of which 67% is derived from complex carbohydrates and naturally occurring sugars, 18% from fats, and 15% from proteins. The protein intake is entirely from plant sources, but still provides approximately 55 grams of protein, an amount well above the recommended daily allowance, or RDA, for someone requiring 1,500 calories. At least one-half of the fat servings should be from nuts, seeds, and other whole foods from list 5, the fats and oils list. The dietary fiber intake is 31 to 74.5 grams. The list that follows summarizes this information.

Percentage of calories as carbohydrates: 67%

Percentage of calories as fats: 18%

Percentage of calories as protein: 15%

Protein content: 55 grams

Dietary fiber content: 31 to 74.5 grams

The remainder of this section presents the other diets of the Healthy Exchange System. Find the one that is right for you.

1,500-Calorie Omnivore Diet (daily intake)

List 1 (vegetables)	5 servings
List 2 (fruits)	2.5 servings
List 3 (breads, cereals, and starchy vegetables)	6 servings
List 4 (legumes)	1 serving
List 5 (fats and oils)	5 servings
List 6 (milk)	1 serving
List 7 (meats, fish, cheese, and eggs)	2 servings

Percentage of calories as carbohydrates: 67%

Percentage of calories as fats: 18%

Percentage of calories as protein: 15%

Protein content: 61 grams (75% from plant sources)

Dietary fiber content: 19.5 to 53.5 grams

2,000-Calorie Vegan Diet (daily intake)

List 1 (vegetables)	5.5 servings
List 2 (fruits)	2 servings
List 3 (breads, cereals, and starchy vegetables)	11 servings
List 4 (legumes)	5 servings
List 5 (fats and oils)	8 servings

Percentage of calories as carbohydrates: 67%

Percentage of calories as fats: 18%

Percentage of calories as protein: 15%

Protein content: 79 grams

Dietary fiber content: 48.5 to 101.5 grams

2,000-Calorie Omnivore Diet (daily intake)

List 1 (vegetables)	5 servings
List 2 (fruits)	2.5 servings
List 3 (breads, cereals, and starchy vegetables)	13 servings
List 4 (legumes)	2 servings
List 5 (fats and oils)	7 servings
List 6 (milk)	1 serving
List 7 (meats, fish, cheese, and eggs)	2 servings

Percentage of calories as carbohydrates: 66%

Percentage of calories as fats: 19%

Percentage of calories as protein: 15%

Protein content: 78 grams (72% from plant sources)

Dietary fiber content: 32.5 to 88.5 grams

2,500-Calorie Vegan Diet (daily intake)

List 1 (vegetables)	8 servings
List 2 (fruits)	3 servings
List 3 (breads, cereals, and starchy vegetables)	17 servings
List 4 (legumes)	5 servings
List 5 (fats and oils)	8 servings

Percentage of calories as carbohydrates: 69%

Percentage of calories as fats: 15%

Percentage of calories as protein: 16%

Protein content: 101 grams

Dietary fiber content: 33 to 121 grams

2,500-Calorie Omnivore Diet (daily intake)

List 1 (vegetables)	8 servings
List 2 (fruits)	3.5 servings

List 3 (breads, cereals, and starchy vegetables)	17 servings
List 4 (legumes)	2 servings
List 5 (fats and oils)	8 servings
List 6 (milk)	1 serving
List 7 (meats, fish, cheese, and eggs)	3 servings

    Percentage of calories as carbohydrates: 66%

    Percentage of calories as fats: 18%

    Percentage of calories as protein: 16%

    Protein content: 102 grams (80% from plant sources)

    Dietary fiber content: 40.5 to 116.5 grams

3,000-Calorie Vegan Diet (daily intake)

List 1 (vegetables)	10 servings
List 2 (fruits)	4 servings
List 3 (breads, cereals, and starchy vegetables)	17 servings
List 4 (legumes)	6 servings
List 5 (fats and oils)	10 servings

    Percentage of calories as carbohydrates: 70%

    Percentage of calories as fats: 16%

    Percentage of calories as protein: 14%

    Protein content: 116 grams

    Dietary fiber content: 50 to 84 grams

3,000-Calorie Omnivore Diet (daily intake)

List 1 (vegetables)	10 servings
List 2 (fruits)	3 servings
List 3 (breads, cereals, and starchy vegetables)	20 servings
List 4 (legumes)	2 servings

List 5 (fats and oils)   10 servings
List 6 (milk)   1 serving
List 7 (meats, fish, cheese, and eggs)   3 servings
Percentage of calories as carbohydrates: 67%
Percentage of calories as fats: 18%
Percentage of calories as protein: 15%
Protein content: 116 grams (81% from plant sources)
Dietary fiber content: 45 to 133 grams

Note: Use these diets as the basis for calculating diets of specific calorie amounts. For example, for a 4,000-calorie diet, add the 2,500-calorie diet to the 1,500-calorie diet. For a 1,000-calorie diet, divide the 2,000-calorie diet in half.

In the next seven sections you will examine each Exchange List in the Healthy Exchange System. You will learn about the general characteristics of each category of food and how individual foods can benefit you or be detrimental to nutrition. In each section, an Exchange List appears. From these lists, each day, you will choose foods to meet the serving requirements defined by your diet.

List 1: Vegetables

Vegetables are excellent sources of vitamins, minerals, and health-promoting fiber compounds. Vegetables are fantastic "diet" foods because they are very high in nutritional value but low in calories.

Please notice that starchy vegetables like potatoes and yams are included in list 3 (breads, cereals, and starchy vegetables). Notice also that list 1 contains a category for "free" vegetables. These vegetables are termed free because you can eat them in any amount desired; the calories they contain are offset by the number of calories your body will burn to digest them. If you are trying to lose weight, these foods are especially valuable because they will help to keep you feeling satisfied between meals.

Because the recommended amounts of vegetables are quite high, you may find it necessary to consume them in the form of fresh juice. Juicing allows for easy absorption of the health-giving properties of vegetables.

Vegetables

Measured-serving vegetables

Unless otherwise noted, 1 serving consists of 1 cup of cooked vegetables or fresh vegetable juice or 2 cups of raw vegetables.

Artichoke (1 medium)

Asparagus

Bean sprouts

Beets

Broccoli

Brussels sprouts

Carrots

Cauliflower

Eggplant

Greens

    Beet

    Chard

    Collard

    Dandelion

    Kale

    Mustard

    Spinach (cooked)

    Turnip

Mushrooms
Okra
Onions
Rhubarb
Rutabaga
Sauerkraut
String beans, green or yellow
Summer squash
Tomatoes, tomato juice, vegetable juice cocktail
Zucchini

Free vegetables
Eat as many of the following items as you wish.

Alfalfa sprouts
Bell peppers
Bok choy
Cabbage
Celery
Chicory
Chinese cabbage
Cucumber
Endive
Escarole
Lettuce
Parsley
Radishes
Spinach
Turnips
Watercress

List 2: Fruits

Fruits make excellent snacks because they contain fructose, or fruit sugar. This sugar is absorbed slowly into the bloodstream, allowing the body time to utilize it. Also, fruits are excellent sources of vitamins and minerals as well as health-promoting fiber compounds and flavonoids. However, fruits are not as beneficial as vegetables, because they tend to be higher in calories. That is why vegetables are favored over fruits in weight-loss plans and healthful diets.

Fruits

Each of the following equals 1 serving.

Fresh fruit and fruit-based items

Fresh juice, 1 cup (8 ounces)*

Pasteurized juice, ⅔ cup

Apple, 1 large

Applesauce (unsweetened), 1 cup

Apricots, dried, 8 halves

Apricots, fresh, 4 medium

Banana, 1 medium

Berries

    Blackberries, 1 cup

    Blueberries, 1 cup

    Cranberries, 1 cup

    Raspberries, 1 cup

    Strawberries, 1½ cups

Cherries, 20 large

Dates, 4

Figs, dried, 2

Figs, fresh, 2

Grapefruit, 1

Grapes, 20

Mango, 1 small

Melons

    Cantaloupe, ½ small

    Honeydew, ¼ medium

    Watermelon, 2 cups

Nectarines, 2 small

Orange, 1 large

Papaya, 1½ cups

Peaches, 2 medium

Persimmons, native, 2 medium

Pineapple, 1 cup

Plums, 4 medium

Prune juice, ½ cup

Prunes, 4 medium

Raisins, 4 tablespoons

Tangerines, 2 medium

Processed fruit and other products

Eat no more than 1 serving of the following "fruit" foods per day.

Honey, 1 tablespoon

Jams, jellies, preserves, 1 tablespoon

Sugar, 1 tablespoon

*Although 1 cup of most fruit juices equals 1 serving, prune juice is an exception; consult the alphabetized portion of the list.

List 3: Breads, Cereals, and Starchy Vegetables

Breads, cereals, and starchy vegetables are classified as complex carbohydrates. Complex carbohydrates are made up of long chains of simple carbohydrates, or sugars. The body has to digest, or break down, the large sugar chains into simple sugars. Therefore, the sugar from complex carbohydrates enters the bloodstream slowly. This means a relatively stable blood sugar level and appetite.

Complex carbohydrates—breads, cereals, and starchy vegetables—are higher in fiber and nutrients but lower in calories than simple-sugar items such as cakes and candies.

Note that some of the prepared foods included in the list of breads, cereals, and starchy vegetables constitute more than 1 serving.

Breads, Cereals, and Starchy Vegetables

Each of the following items equals 1 serving.

> Breads
>
> Bagel, small, ½
>
> Dinner roll, 1
>
> Dried bread crumbs, 3 tablespoons
>
> English muffin, small, ½
>
> Tortilla (6 inch), 1
>
> Whole wheat, rye, or pumpernickel, 1 slice

Cereals

> Bran flakes, ½ cup
>
> Cornmeal (dry), 2 tablespoons
>
> Flour, 2½ tablespoons
>
> Grits (cooked), ½ cup
>
> Pasta (cooked), ½ cup
>
> Porridge (cooked cereal), ½ cup
>
> Puffed cereal (unsweetened), 1 cup
>
> Rice or barley (cooked), ½ cup
>
> Unpuffed unsweetened cereal, ¾ cup
>
> Wheat germ, ¼ cup

Crackers

    Arrowroot, 3

    Graham (2½-inch squares), 2

    Matzo (4 by 6 inches), ½

    Rye wafers (2 by 3½ inches), 3

    Saltine, 6

Starchy vegetables

    Corn, kernels, ⅓ cup

    Corn on the cob, 1 small cob

    Parsnips, ⅔ cup

    Potato, mashed, ½ cup

    Potato, white, 1 small

    Squash (acorn, butternut, or winter), ½ cup

    Yam or sweet potato, ¼ cup

Prepared foods

Each of the following items equals 1 "bread" serving, but you must omit 1 or more fat servings to maintain the nutrition balance of your diet.

    Biscuit, 2-inch diameter, 1 (omit 1 fat serving)

    Corn bread, 2 by 2 by 1 inch, 1 (omit 1 fat serving)

    French fries, 2 to 3 inches long, 8 (omit 1 fat serving)

    Muffin, small, 1 (omit 1 fat serving)

    Pancake, 5 by ½ inch, 1 (omit 1 fat serving)

    Potato or corn chips, 15 (omit 2 fat servings)

    Waffle, 5 by ½ inch, 1 (omit 1 fat serving)

List 4: Legumes

According to the dictionary, a legume is a plant that produces a pod that splits on both sides. Of the common human foods, beans, peas, lentils, and peanuts are legumes. The legume category also includes alfalfa, clover, acacia, and indigo.

Legumes are fantastic foods because they are rich in important nutrients and health-promoting compounds. Legumes help improve liver function, lower cholesterol levels, and improve blood sugar control. Since obesity and diabetes have been linked to loss of blood sugar control (insulin insensitivity), legumes appear to be extremely important in weight-loss plans and in the dietary management of diabetes.

Legumes

In this list, ½ cup of each item, cooked or sprouted, equals 1 serving.

Black-eyed peas

Chickpeas

Garbanzo beans

Kidney beans

Lentils

Lima beans

Pinto beans

Soybeans, including tofu (omit 1 fat serving)

Split peas

Other dried beans and peas

List 5: Fats and Oils

As stated earlier, typical animal fats are solid at room temperature and are referred to as saturated fats; vegetable fats are liquid at room temperature and are referred to as unsaturated fats or unsaturated oils. Vegetable oils provide the greatest source of the essential fatty acids linoleic acid and linolenic acid. These fatty acids function in our bodies as components of nerve cells, cellular membranes, and hormonelike substances. Fats also provide the body with energy.

Fats are important to human health, but too much fat in the diet, especially saturated fat, is linked to numerous cancers, heart disease, and stroke. Most nutrition experts strongly recommend that you keep total fat intake to below 30% of total calories. They recommend also that you consume at least twice as much unsaturated fat as saturated fat.

Fats and Oils

Each of the following items equals 1 serving.

Mono-unsaturated

Olive oil, 1 teaspoon

Olives, 5 small

Polyunsaturated

Almonds, 10 whole

Avocado (4-inch diameter), ⅛ fruit

Peanuts

    Spanish, 20 whole

    Virginia, 10 whole

Pecans, 2 large

Seeds

    Flax, 1 tablespoon

    Pumpkin, 1 tablespoon

    Sesame, 1 tablespoon

    Sunflower, 1 tablespoon

Vegetable oil

    Canola, 1 teaspoon

    Corn, 1 teaspoon

    Flaxseed, 1 teaspoon

    Safflower, 1 teaspoon

Soy, 1 teaspoon

Sunflower, 1 teaspoon

Walnuts, 6 small

Saturated (use sparingly)

Bacon, 1 slice

Butter, 1 teaspoon

Cream, heavy, 1 tablespoon

Cream, light or sour, 2 tablespoons

Cream cheese, 1 tablespoon

Mayonnaise, 1 teaspoon

Salad dressing, 2 teaspoons

List 6: Milk

Is milk for everybody? Definitely not. Many people are allergic to milk or lack the enzymes necessary to digest it. The drinking of cow's milk is a relatively new dietary practice for humans. This may be the reason so many people have difficulty with milk. Limit milk consumption to no more than 2 servings per day.

Milk

For each of the following items, 1 cup equals 1 "milk" serving, but for some items you must omit 1 or more fat servings to maintain the nutrition balance of your diet.

Nonfat milk or yogurt

Nonfat soy milk

2% milk or soy milk (omit 1 fat serving)

Lowfat yogurt (omit 1 fat serving)

Whole milk (omit 2 fat servings)

Yogurt (omit 2 fat servings)

List 7: Meats, Fish, Cheese, and Eggs

When choosing from this list, choose primarily from the lowfat group and remove the skin of poultry. This practice will keep the amount of saturated fat low. List 7 provides high concentrations of certain nutrients difficult to get in an entirely vegetarian diet. It provides the full range of amino acids, vitamin B12, and heme iron. Nonetheless, if you have rheumatoid arthritis, it is best to avoid the meat food group with the exception of cold-water fish.

Meats, Fish, Cheese, and Eggs

Each of the following items equals 1 serving.

Lowfat items

Beef, 1 ounce

> Baby beef, chipped beef, chuck, round (bottom, top), rump (all cuts), spareribs, steak (flank, plate), tenderloin plate ribs, tripe

Cottage cheese, lowfat, ¼ cup

Fish, 1 ounce

Lamb, 1 ounce

> Leg, loin (roast and chops), ribs, shank, shoulder, sirloin

Poultry (chicken or turkey without skin), 1 ounce

Veal, 1 ounce

> Cutlet, leg, loin, rib, shank, shoulder

Medium-fat items

For each of the following items, omit ½ fat serving.

Beef, 1 ounce

> Canned corned beef, ground (15% fat), rib eye, round (ground commercial)

Cheese, 1 ounce

> Farmer, Mozzarella, Parmesan, ricotta

Eggs, 1

Organ meats, 1 ounce

Peanut butter, 2 tablespoons

Pork, 1 ounce

> Boiled, Boston butt, Canadian bacon, loin (all tender-loin), picnic

High-fat items

For each of the following items, omit 2 fat servings.

Beef, 1 ounce

> Brisket, corned beef, ground beef (more than 20% fat), hamburger, roasts (rib), steaks (club and rib)

Cheese, cheddar, 1 ounce

Duck or goose, 1 ounce

Lamb, breast, 1 ounce

Pork, 1 ounce

> Country-style ham, deviled ham, ground pork, loin, spareribs

Menu Planning

The Healthy Exchange System was created to ensure that you are consuming a diet that provides adequate nutrients in their proper ratio. These exchange recommendations will help you a great deal in constructing a daily menu—and so will the recipes you will find in the following pages.

Breakfast

Breakfast is an absolute must. Healthful breakfast choices include whole-grain cereals, muffins, and breads, along with fresh whole fruit or fresh fruit juice. Cereals, both hot and cold and preferably from whole grains, may be the best food choices for breakfast. The complex carbohydrates in the grains provide sustained energy. An evaluation of data from the National Health and Nutrition Examination Survey II (a national survey of the nutrition and health practices of Americans) disclosed that blood cholesterol levels are lowest among adults who eat whole-grain cereal for breakfast. Individuals who consumed other breakfast foods had blood cholesterol levels higher than those of the whole-grain cereal eaters. Cholesterol levels were highest among those who typically skipped breakfast.

Here is a simple, yet nutritious, way to start off a healthful day.

Hot Cereal

Makes 2 servings

5	cups water
2	cups rolled oats
½	teaspoon vanilla (*optional*)
4	tablespoons honey
¼	teaspoon cinnamon (*optional*)
½	teaspoon flaxseed oil

In a medium saucepan, combine the water and oats. Cook, covered, over medium heat until the mixture is bubbling (about 5 minutes). Reduce heat and remove cover. Stirring occasionally, simmer uncovered until the oats are soft (about 15 minutes). For a creamier cereal, simmer for 5 minutes longer. Remove from heat and add vanilla, honey, cinnamon, and flaxseed oil. Pour into bowls.

Dietary Servings Per Recipe Serving
Fruits: ½
Grains and starches: 1
Fats: ½

Nutrition Information Per Recipe Serving
Calories: 140
Carbohydrate: 70%
Protein: 14%
Fat: 16%
Fiber: 1.6 grams
Calcium: 31 milligrams

Instead of honey, you can add one sliced banana, ½ cup raisins, or ½ cup fruit juice.

Lunch

Lunch is a great time to enjoy a healthful bowl of soup, a large salad, and some whole-grain bread. Bean soups and other legume dishes are especially good lunch selections for people with diabetes and blood sugar problems; these selections can improve blood sugar regulation. Legumes are filling, yet low in calories.

Black-Bean Soup

Makes 4 servings

2	teaspoons extra-virgin olive oil *or* canola oil
2	medium red onions, chopped
1	jalapeño chile, minced
2	large garlic cloves, minced
1	teaspoon ground cumin
½	teaspoon chili powder
2	cups water
4	cups cooked black beans
2	tablespoons sour cream (*optional*)

In a medium saucepan, heat olive oil. Add onion and chile. Cook over moderate heat, stirring frequently, until onion begins to brown (about 4 minutes). Stir in garlic. Reduce heat to low and cook, stirring constantly, for 1 minute. Stir in cumin and chili powder. Remove from heat. In a large heavy pot, place the water, beans, and spice mixture. Cook over low heat, stirring occasionally, until beans are hot (about 5 minutes). If a smooth texture is preferred, transfer the soup to a food processor or blender and purée before serving. Top each serving with sour cream.

Dietary Servings Per Recipe Serving
Vegetables: 1
Legumes: 2
Fats: ½

Nutrition Information Per Recipe Serving
Calories: 248
Carbohydrate: 65%
Protein: 19%
Fat: 16%
Fiber: 22 grams
Calcium: 137 milligrams

This soup can be made up to four days ahead. Simply refrigerate it in an airtight container, then reheat the soup when you're ready.

Herb Dressing

Makes 8 servings (2 tablespoons per serving)

6   tablespoons vegetable oil
2   teaspoons chopped fresh parsley

2 teaspoons chopped fresh chives
2 tablespoons chopped fresh chervil *or* 2 teaspoons dried chervil
   Black pepper, to taste
½ cup rice vinegar
2 tablespoons water
3 cloves garlic, minced
2 teaspoons dried mustard

In a blender, combine all ingredients. Blend thoroughly.

Snacks

The best snacks are nuts, seeds, and fresh fruit and vegetables.

Dinner

For dinner, the most healthful meals contain a fresh vegetable salad, a cooked vegetable side dish or a bowl of soup, whole grains, and legumes. The whole grains may be provided in bread or pasta, as a side dish, or in an entrée. The legumes can be in soups, salads, and main dishes.

Although a varied diet rich in whole grains, vegetables, and legumes can provide optimal levels of protein, many people like to eat meat. The important thing is not to over-consume animal products. Limit your intake to no more than 6 ounces per day, and choose fish, skinless poultry, and lean cuts rather than fat-ladened choices. If you have rheumatoid arthritis, you are better off avoiding meat altogether.

Here is a recipe from *The Healing Power of Foods Cookbook* (Michael T. Murray, Prima Publishing, Rocklin, CA, 1993) that is a great alternative to Beef Stroganoff and provides a complete-protein meal from vegetable sources.

Mushroom Stroganoff with Tofu

Makes 4 servings

Stroganoff

1	teaspoon canola oil *or* olive oil
½	onion, minced
1	clove garlic, minced (*optional*)
1	pound fresh mushrooms, sliced
4	ounces tofu
1	teaspoon oregano
2	cups cooked brown rice
1	tablespoon toasted slivered almonds
1	tablespoon chopped fresh parsley

Sauce

8	ounces tofu
¼	cup water
2	tablespoons soy sauce
2	tablespoons lemon juice *or* apple cider vinegar
1	clove garlic
1	teaspoon chopped ginger root

Make the sauce first. Then select a large skillet in which to make the stroganoff. Heat oil. Over medium heat sauté onion and garlic until onion is transparent. Add mushrooms; sauté until slightly limp and moisture has evaporated. Set aside. Cut tofu into 1-inch cubes. Add tofu to skillet and brown cubes slightly. Pour sauce over all. Mix well and heat through, stirring. Blend in oregano. Serve over brown rice (½ cup per person) and sprinkle with almonds and parsley.

Sauce   Place all ingredients in a blender. Blend until very smooth. Be sure garlic and ginger root are well chopped; no chunks should remain. Set sauce aside for use within a few hours; refrigerate if use will be significantly delayed. (Refrigeration improves flavor.) Refrigerated, the sauce will keep up to one week.

Dietary Servings Per Recipe Serving
Vegetables: ½
Grains and Starches: 1
Legumes: 1
Fats: ½

Nutrition Information Per Recipe Serving
Calories: 208
Carbohydrate: 56%
Protein: 21%
Fat: 23%
Fiber: 3 grams
Calcium: 160 milligrams

Food Allergies

In addition to the guidelines of the Healthy Exchange System, people with rheumatoid arthritis need to be concerned about food allergies. An allergy occurs when the body reacts adversely to the ingestion of a food. The reaction may or may not be mediated by the immune system. The reaction may be caused by a protein, starch, or other food component or by a contaminant found in the food (colorings, preservatives, and the like). A classic food allergy occurs when an ingested food molecule acts as an antigen, or a substance that can be bound by an antibody. The antibodies that do the binding are known as IgE (pronounced "eye-gee-ee"). IgE then binds to specialized white blood cells known as mast cells and basophils. This binding causes the release of substances such as histamine, which cause swelling and inflammation.

Other words often used to refer to a food allergy include *food hypersensitivity, food anaphylaxis, food idiosyncrasy, food intolerance, pharmacologic* (or *druglike*) *reaction to food, metabolic reaction to food,* and *food sensitivity.*

The number of people suffering from food allergies has increased dramatically during the last 15 years. Some physicians claim that food allergies are the leading cause of most undiagnosed symptoms and that at least 60% of Americans suffer from symptoms associated with food reactions. Theories of why the incidence has increased include increased stresses on the immune system (such as greater chemical pollution in the air, water, and food); earlier weaning and earlier introduction of solid foods to infants; genetic manipulation of plants, resulting in food components with greater allergenic tendencies; and increased ingestion of fewer foods. Probably all of these and more have contributed to the increased frequency and severity of food allergy symptoms.

Signs and Symptoms of Food Allergies

Food allergies have been implicated as a causative factor in a wide range of conditions.[4,5] The actual symptoms produced during an allergic response depend on the location of the immune system activation, the mediators of inflammation involved, and the sensitivity of the tissues to specific mediators. Table 7.4 presents a summary of common symptoms of food allergy.

Identification of Food Allergies

Although laboratory tests can identify food allergies, many physicians believe that oral food challenge is the best way of diagnosing adverse reactions to foods. The most popular challenge method involves using an elimination diet. The patient is placed on a limited diet; commonly eaten foods are eliminated and replaced with either hypoallergenic foods

Table 7.4 Symptoms and Diseases Commonly Associated with Food Allergy

System or Part of Body	Symptoms or Diseases
Gastrointestinal	Canker sores, celiac disease, chronic diarrhea, stomach ulcer, gas, gastritis, irritable colon, malabsorption, ulcerative colitis
Genitourinary	Bedwetting, chronic bladder infection, kidney disease
Immune	Chronic infection, especially ear infections
Brain	Anxiety, depression, hyperactivity, inability to concentrate, insomnia, irritability, confusion, personality change, seizures
Musculoskeletal	Bursitis, joint pain, low back pain
Respiratory	Asthma, chronic bronchitis, wheezing
Skin	Acne, eczema, hives, itching, skin rash
Miscellaneous	Irregular heartbeat; edema, fainting; fatigue; headaches, especially migraines; hypoglycemia; itchy nose or throat; sinusitis

and foods rarely eaten, or special hypoallergenic meal replacement formulas. The standard elimination diet (also known as an oligoiantigenic diet) consists of lamb, chicken, potatoes, rice, banana, apple, and a cabbage-family vegetable (cabbage, Brussels sprouts, broccoli, and the like). (In the treatment of rheumatoid arthritis, the best elimination diet may be the one employed in the study detailed on page 58). In this study, treatment began with a therapeutic fast for 7 to 10 days.[6] Dietary intake during the fast consisted of herbal teas; garlic; vegetable broth; decoction of potatoes and parsley; and juices made from carrots, beets, or celery.

After the elimination diet or fast, individual foods are reintroduced. A "new" food item is added to the diet every second day. Reintroduction of a problem food will typically produce a more severe or recognizable symptom than it did before. The patient must keep a careful, detailed record describing when foods were reintroduced and what symptoms appeared upon reintroduction. If a food seems to cause an increase in pain, stiffness, or joint swelling within 2 to 48 hours of reintroduction, the patient omits that food from the diet for at least 7 days before reintroducing it a second time. If the food again causes worsening of symptoms, it should probably be omitted permanently from the diet.

Management of Food Allergies

Once you have determined the food that is causing an allergy, the simplest and most effective method of dealing with it is through avoidance. Avoidance means not only avoiding the food in its most identifiable state (for example, eggs in an omelette), but also in its hidden state (for example, eggs in bread). You may need to eliminate foods that are closely related to the problem food or other foods containing components similar to it. (Patients with severe wheat allergy might have to avoid rice and millet, for example.) It is also important to eliminate food additives.

Food additives are used to prevent spoiling or enhance flavor and include such substances as preservatives, artificial colors, artificial flavorings, and acidifiers. The U.S. Food and Drug Administration has approved the use of over 2,800 different food additives. Although the government has banned many synthetic food additives, do not assume that all the additives currently used in our food supply are safe. There are still a great number of synthetic food additives still in use that are being linked to allergies and such diseases as depression, asthma, hyperactivity and learning disabilities in children, and migraine headaches.[4]

If a person has multiple food allergies, a rotary diversified diet is the best method of eating to follow. This diet consists of eating a highly varied selection of foods in a definite order.

This prevents the formation of new allergies and controls pre-existing ones. Tolerated foods are eaten at regularly spaced intervals of four to seven days. For example, if a man has wheat on Monday, he will have to wait until Friday to have anything with wheat in it again. This approach is based on the principle that infrequent consumption of tolerated foods is not likely to induce new allergies or increase any mild allergies. As tolerance for eliminated foods returns, they may be added back into the rotation schedule without reactivation of the allergy. (This applies, of course, only to cyclic food allergies. Fixed allergenic foods may never be eaten again.)

Following the Rotary Diversified Diet is not simply a matter of rotating tolerated foods; food families must also be rotated. Foods, whether animal or vegetable, come in families. Foods in one family can cross-react with allergy-inducing foods. Steady consumption of foods of the same family can lead to allergies. Food families need not be as strictly rotated as individual foods. It is usually recommended to avoid eating members of the same food family two days in a row. Table 7.5 lists family classifications for edible plants and animals. Table 7.6 presents a simplified four-day rotation diet plan.

Final Comments

I firmly believe that the quality of one's life is directly related to the quality of the foods one routinely ingests. The human body is the most remarkable machine in the world, but most Americans are not feeding the body the high-quality fuel it deserves. When a machine does not receive the proper fuel or maintenance, how long can it be expected to run in an efficient manner? If your body is not fed the full range of nutrients it needs, how can it be expected to stay in a state of good health?

Table 7.5   Taxonomic List of Edible Plants and Animals*

Vegetables

Legumes	**Mustard**	**Parsley**	**Potato**
Beans	Broccoli	Anise	Chile
Cocoa beans	Brussels sprouts	Caraway	Eggplant
Lentils	Cabbage	Carrot	Peppers
Licorice	Cauliflower	Celery	Potatoes
Peanuts	Mustard	Coriander	Tobacco
Peas	Radish	Cumin	Tomato
Soybeans	Turnip	Parsley	
Tamarinds	Watercress		

Grass	**Lily**	**Laurel**	**Sunflower**
Barley	Asparagus	Avocado	Artichoke
Corn	Chives	Camphor	Lettuce
Oat	Garlic	Cinnamon	Sunflower
Rice	Leeks		
Rye	Onions		
Wheat			

Beet	**Buckwheat**
Beet	Buckwheat
Chard	Rhubarb
Spinach	

Fruits

Gourds	**Plums**	**Citrus**	**Cashew**
Cantaloupe	Almond	Grapefruit	Cashews
Cucumber	Apricot	Lemon	Mango
Honeydew	Cherry	Lime	Pistachio
Melons	Peach	Mandarin	
Pumpkin	Persimmon	Orange	
Squash	Plum	Tangerine	
Zucchini			

Table 7.5 *(continued)*

Fruits (cont.)

Nuts	**Beech**	**Banana**	**Palm**
Brazil nuts	Beechnuts	Arrowroot	Coconut
Pecans	Chestnuts	Banana	Date
Walnuts	Chinquapin nuts	Plantain	Date sugar

Grape	**Pineapple**	**Rose**	**Birch**
Grape	Pineapple	Blackberry	Filberts
Raisin		Loganberry	Hazelnuts
		Raspberry	
		Rose hips	
		Strawberry	

Apple	**Blueberry**	**Pawpaws**
Apple	Blueberry	Papaya
Pear	Cranberry	Pawpaw
Quince	Huckleberry	

Animals

Mammals (Meat/Milk)	**Birds (Meat/Egg)**	**Fish**	
Cow	Chicken	Catfish	Salmon
Goat	Duck	Cod	Sardine
Pig	Goose	Flounder	Snapper
Rabbit	Hen	Halibut	Trout
Sheep	Turkey	Mackerel	Tuna

Crustaceans	**Mollusks**
Crab	Abalone
Crayfish	Clams
Lobster	Mussels
Prawn	Oysters
Shrimp	Scallops

*The names of food families are shown in this table in boldface.

Table 7.6   The Four-Day Rotation Diet

Food Family	Food
Day 1	
Citrus	Lemon, orange, grapefruit, lime, tangerine, kumquat, citron
Banana	Banana, plantain, arrowroot (musa)
Palm	Coconut, date, date sugar
Parsley	Carrots, parsnips, celery, celery seed, celeriac, anise, dill, fennel, cumin, parsley, coriander, caraway
Spices	Black and white pepper, peppercorn, nutmeg, mace
Subucaya	Brazil nuts
Bird	All fowl and game birds, including chicken, turkey, duck, goose, guinea, pigeon, quail, pheasant, eggs
Juices	Juices (preferably fresh) may be made and used from any fruits and vegetables listed above, in any combination desired, without adding sweeteners.
Day 2	
Grape	All varieties of grapes, raisins
Pineapple	Juice-pack, water-pack, or fresh
Rose	Strawberry, raspberry, blackberry, loganberry, rose hips
Gourd	Watermelon, cucumber, cantaloupe, pumpkin, squash, other melons, zucchini, pumpkin or squash seeds
Beet	Beet, spinach, chard
Legume	Pea, black-eyed pea, dry beans, green beans, carob, soybeans, lentils, licorice, peanut, alfalfa
Cashew	Cashew, pistachio, mango
Birch	Filberts, hazelnuts
Flaxseed	Flaxseed
Swine	All pork products
Mollusks	Abalone, snail, squid, clam, mussel, oyster, scallop
Crustaceans	Crab, crayfish, lobster, prawn, shrimp
Juices	Juices (preferably fresh) may be made and used without added sweeteners from any fruits, berries, or vegetables listed above, in any combination desired, including fresh alfalfa and some legumes.

Table 7.6   *(continued)*

Food Family	Food
Day 3	
Apple	Apple, pear, quince
Gooseberry	Currant, gooseberry
Buckwheat	Buckwheat, rhubarb
Aster	Lettuce, chicory, endive, escarole, globe artichoke, dandelion, sunflower seeds, tarragon
Potato	Potato, tomato, eggplant, peppers (red and green), chile pepper, paprika, cayenne, ground cherries
Lily (onion)	Onion, garlic, asparagus, chives, leeks
Spurge	Tapioca
Herb	Basil, savory, sage, oregano, horehound, catnip, spearmint, peppermint, thyme, marjoram, lemon balm
Walnut	English walnut, black walnut, pecan, hickory nut, butternut
Pedalium	Sesame
Beech	Chestnut
Saltwater fish	Herring, anchovy, cod, sea bass, sea trout, mackerel, tuna, swordfish, flounder, sole
Freshwater fish	Sturgeon, salmon, whitefish, bass, perch
Juices	Juices (preferably fresh) may be made and used without added sweeteners from any fruits and vegetables listed above, in any combination.
Day 4	
Plum	Plum, cherry, peach, apricot, nectarine, almond, wild cherry
Blueberry	Blueberry, huckleberry, cranberry, wintergreen
Pawpaws	Pawpaw, papaya, papain
Mustard	Mustard, turnip, radish, horseradish, watercress, cabbage, Chinese cabbage, broccoli, cauliflower, Brussels sprouts, kale, kohlrabi, rutabaga
Laurel	Avocado, cinnamon, bay leaf, sassafras, cassia buds or bark
Sweet potato or yam	

Table 7.6 *(continued)*

Food Family	Food
Day 4 (cont.)	
Grass	Wheat, corn, rice, oats, barley, rye, wild rice, cane, millet, sorghum, bamboo sprouts
Orchid	Vanilla
Protea	Macadamia nut
Conifer	Pine nut
Fungus	Mushrooms and yeast (brewer's yeast, etc.)
Bovid	Milk products—butter, cheese, yogurt, beef and milk products, oleomargarine, lamb
Juices	Juices (preferably fresh) may be made and used without added sweeteners from any fruits and vegetables listed above, in any combination desired.

References

Preface

Ortus WJ and Stone A: The addiction to drug companies. Biological Psychiatry 32:847–9, 1992.

Chapter 1: What Is Osteoarthritis?

1. Bland JH and Cooper SM: Osteoarthritis: A review of the cell biology involved and evidence for reversibility. Management rationally related to known genesis and pathophysiology. Semin Arthr Rheum 14:106–33, 1984.

2. Perry GH, Smith MJG, and Whiteside CG: Spontaneous recovery of the hip joint space in degenerative hip disease. Ann Rheum Dis 31:440–8, 1972.

3. Brooks PM, Potter SR, and Buchanan WW: NSAID and osteoarthritis—help or hindrance. J Rheumatol 9:3–5, 1982.

4. Shield MJ: Anti-inflammatory drugs and their effects on cartilage synthesis and renal function. Eur J Rheum Inflam 13:7–16, 1993.

5. Newman NM and Ling RSM: Acetabular bone destruction related to non-steroidal anti-inflammatory drugs. Lancet ii:11–3, 1985.

6. Solomon L: Drug induced arthropathy and necrosis of the femoral head. J Bone Joint Surg 55B:246–51, 1973.

7. Ronningen H and Langeland N: Indomethacin treatment in osteo-arthritis of the hip joint. Acta Orthop Scand 50:169–74, 1979.

Chapter 2: The Natural Approach to Osteoarthritis

1. Sullivan MX and Hess WC: Cystine content of finger nails in arthritis. J Bone Joint Surg 16:185–8, 1935.

2. Senturia BD: Results of treatment of chronic arthritis and rheuma-toid conditions with colloidal sulphur. J Bone Joint Surg 16:119–25, 1934.

3. Childers NF: A Diet to Stop Arthritis. Somerset Press, Somerville, NJ, 1991.

4. Setnikar I, Pacini A, and Revel L: Antiarthritic effects of gluco-samine sulfate studied in animal models. Arzneim-Forsch 41: 542–5, 1991.

5. Vaz AL: Double-blind clinical evaluation of the relative efficacy of ibuprofen and glucosamine sulfate in the management of osteo-arthrosis of the knee in out-patients. Current Med Res Opin 8:145–9, 1982.

6. Crolle G and D'este E: Glucosamine sulfate for the management of arthrosis: A controlled clinical investigation. Current Med Res Opin 7:104–14, 1981.

7. Tapadinhas MJ, Rivera IC, and Bignamini AA: Oral glucosamine sul-fate in the management of arthrosis: Report on a multi-centre open investigation in Portugal. Pharmatherapeutica 3:157–68, 1982.

8. D'Ambrosia ED, Casa B, Bompani R, et al.: Glucosamine sulphate: A controlled clinical investigation in arthrosis. Pharmatherapeutica 2:504–8, 1982.

9. Vaz AL: Double-blind clinical evaluation of the relative efficacy of ibuprofen and glucosamine sulfate in the management of osteo-arthrosis of the knee in out-patients. Current Med Res Opin 8:145–9, 1982.

10. Setnikar I, Pacini A, and Revel L: Antiarthritic effects of glucosamine sulfate studied in animal models. Arzneim-Forsch 41: 542–5, 1991.

11. Morrison M: Therapeutic applications of chondroitin-4-sulfate, appraisal of biologic properties. Folia Angiol 25:225–32, 1977.

12. Setnikar I, Giachetti C, and Zanolo G: Pharmacokinetics of glucosamine in the dog and in man. Arzneim-Forsch 36:729–35, 1986.

13. Rejholec V: Long-term studies of antiosteoarthritic drugs: An assessment. Semin Arthr Rheum 17: supplement 1:35–53, 1987.

14. Larkin JG, Capell HA, and Sturrock RD: Seatone in rheumatoid arthritis: A six month placebo-controlled study. Ann Rheum Dis 44:199–201, 1985.

15. Schwartz ER: The modulation of osteoarthritic development by vitamins C and E. Int J Vit Nutr Res (supplement) 26:141–6, 1984.

16. Bates CJ: Proline and hydroxyproline excretion and vitamin C status in elderly human subjects. Clinical Sci Molecular Med 52:535–43, 1977.

17. Krystal G, Morris GM, and Sokoloff L: Stimulation of DNA synthesis by ascorbate in cultures of articular chondrocytes. Arthr Rheum 25:318–25, 1982.

18. Machtey I and Ouaknine L: Tocopherol in osteoarthritis: A controlled pilot study. J Am Geri Soc 26:328–30, 1978.

19. Kaufman W: The use of vitamin therapy to reverse certain concomitants of aging. J Am Geri Soc 3:927, 1955.

20. Hoffer A: Treatment of arthritis by nicotinic acid and nicotinamide. Can Med Assoc J 81:235–9, 1959.

21. Anand JC: Osteoarthritis and pantothenic acid. J Coll Gen Pract 5:136–7, 1963.

22. Anand JC: Osteoarthritis and pantothenic acid. Lancet ii:1168, 1963.

23. General Practitioner Research Group: Calcium pantothenate in arthritis conditions. Practitioner 224:208–11, 1980.

24. Travers RL, Rennie GC, and Newnham RE: Boron and arthritis: The results of a double-blind pilot study. J Nutr Med 1:127–32, 1990.

25. Tsai CL, Liu TK, and Chen TJ: Estrogen and osteoarthritis: A study of synovial estradiol and estradiol receptor binding in human osteoarthritic knees. Biochemical Biophys Res Commun 183: 1287–91, 1992.

26. Singh GB and Atal CK: Pharmacology of an extract of salai guggal ex-*Boswellia serrata,* a new non-steroidal anti-inflammatory agent. Agents Action 18:407–12, 1986.

27. Reddy CK, Chandrakasan G, and Dhar SC: Studies on the metabolism of glycosaminoglycans under the influence of new herbal anti-inflammatory agents. Biochemical Pharmacol 20:3527–34, 1989.

28. Kulkani RR, Patki PS, Jog VP, et al.: Treatment of osteoarthritis with a herbomineral formulation: A double-blind, placebo-controlled, cross-over study. J Ethnopharmacol 33:91–5, 1991.

29. Lanhers MC, Fleurentin J, Mortier F, et al.: Anti-inflammatory and analgesic effects of an aqueous extract of *Harpagophytum procumbens.* Planta Medica 58:117–23, 1992.

30. Whitehouse LW, Znamirowski M, and Paul CJ: Devil's claw (*Harpagophytum procumbens*): No evidence for anti-inflammatory activity in the treatment of arthritic disease. Can Med Assoc J 129:249–51, 1983.

31. McLeod DW, Revell P, and Robinson BV: Investigations of *Harpagophytum procumbens* (devil's claw) in the treatment of experimental inflammation and arthritis in the rat. Br J Pharmacol 66:140P–141P, 1979.

32. Rees WDW, Rhodes J, Wright JE, et al.: Effect of deglycyrrhizinated liquorice on gastric mucosal damage by aspirin. Scand J Gastroent 14:605–7, 1979.

33. Morgan Ag, McAdam WAF, Pacsoo C, et al.: Comparison between cimetidine and Caved-S in the treatment of gastric ulceration, and subsequent maintenance therapy. Gut 23:545–51, 1982.

34. Kassir ZA: Endoscopic controlled trial of four drug regimens in the treatment of chronic duodenal ulceration. Irish Med J 78:153–6, 1985.

Chapter 3: What Is Gout?

1. Petersdorf R, et al. (eds): Harrison's Principles of Internal Medicine. McGraw-Hill, New York, 1983.

2. Long JW: The Essential Guide to Prescription Drugs. Harper Collins, New York, 1992.

Chapter 4: The Natural Approach to Gout

1. Faller J and Fox IH: Ethanol-induced hyperuricemia. N Engl J Med 307:1598–602, 1982.

2. Blau LW: Cherry diet control for gout and arthritis. Texas Report on Biol and Med 8:309–11, 1950.

3. Bindoli A, Valente M, and Cavallini L: Inhibitory action of quercetin on xanthine oxidase and xanthine dehydrogenase activity. Pharm Res Comm 17:831–9, 1985.

4. Busse WW, Kopp DE, and Middleton E: Flavonoid modulation of human neutrophil function. J Allergy Clin Immunol 73:801–9, 1984.

5. Lewis AS, Murphy L, McCalla C, et al.: Inhibition of mammalian xanthine oxidase by folate compounds and amethopterin. J Biol Chem 259:12–5, 1984.

6. Oster KA: Xanthine oxidase and folic acid. Ann Int Med 87:252, 1977.

7. Brady LR, Tyler VE, and Robbers JE: Pharmacognosy, 8th edition. Lea & Febiger, Philadelphia, 1981.

8. Ball GV and Sorensen LB: Pathogenesis of hyperuricemia in saturnine gout. N Engl J Med 280:1199–1202, 1969.

Chapter 5: What Is Rheumatoid Arthritis?

1. Petersdorf R, et al. (eds): Harrison's Principles of Internal Medicine. McGraw-Hill, New York, 1983.

2. Smith MD, Gibson RA, and Brooks PM: Abnormal bowel permeability in ankylosing spondylitis and rheumatoid arthritis. J Rheumatol 12:299–305, 1985.

3. Zaphiropoulos GC: Rheumatoid arthritis and the gut. Br J Rheumatol 25:138–40, 1986.

4. Segal AW, Isenberg DA, Hajirousou V, et al.: Preliminary evidence for gut involvement in the pathogenesis of rheumatoid arthritis. Br J Rheumatol 25:162–6, 1986.

5. Philips PE: Seminars in arthritis and rheumatism: Infectious agents in the pathogenesis of rheumatoid arthritis. Semin Arthr Rheum 16:1–100, 1986.

6. Jenkins R, Rooney P, Jones D, et al.: Increased intestinal permeability in patients with rheumatoid arthritis: A side effect of oral non-steroidal anti-inflammatory drug therapy? Br J Rheum 26:103–7, 1987.

7. Fries JF, Miller SR, Spitz PW, et al.: Toward an epidemiology of gastropathy associated with nonsteroidal antiinflammatory drug use. Gastroenterol 96:647–55, 1989.

8. Scott DL, Coulton BL, Symmons DPM, et al.: Long-term outcome of treating rheumatoid arthritis: Results after 20 years. Lancet i:1108–11, 1989.

Chapter 6: The Natural Approach to Rheumatoid Arthritis

1. Trowell H and Burkitt D: Western Diseases: Their Emergence and Prevention. Harvard University Press, Cambridge, MA, 1981.

2. Darlington LG and Ramsey NW: Clinical review. Review of dietary therapy for rheumatoid arthritis. Br J Rheumatol 32:507–14, 1993.

3. Buchanan HM, Preston SJ, Brooks PM, et al.: Is diet important in rheumatoid arthritis? Br J Rheumatol 30:125–34, 1991.

4. McCrae F, Veerapen K, and Dieppe P: Diet and arthritis. Practitioner 230:359–61, 1986.

5. Darlington LG, Ramsey NW, and Mansfield JR: Placebo-controlled, blind study of dietary manipulation therapy in rheumatoid arthritis. Lancet i:236–8, 1986.

6. Hicklin JA, McEwen LM, and Morgan JE: The effect of diet in rheumatoid arthritis. Clin Allergy 10:463–7, 1980.

7. Panush RS: Delayed reactions to foods. Food allergy and rheumatic disease. Ann Allergy 56:500–3, 1986.

8. Van de Laar MAFJ and Ander Korst JK: Food intolerance in rheumatoid arthritis. I. A double-blind, controlled trial of the clinical effects of elimination of milk allergens and azo dyes. Ann Rheum Dis 51:298–302, 1992.

9. Kjeldsen-Kragh J, Haugen M, Borchgrevink CF, et al.: Controlled trial of fasting and one-year vegetarian diet in rheumatoid arthritis. Lancet 338:899–902, 1991.

10. Skoldstam L, Larsson L, and Lindstrom FD: Effects of fasting and lactovegetarian diet on rheumatoid arthritis. Scand J Rheumatol 8:249–55, 1979.

11. Kroker GP, Stroud RM, Marshall RT, et al.: Fasting and rheumatoid arthritis: A multicenter study. Clin Ecol 2:137–44, 1984.

12. Hafstrom I, Ringertz B, Gyllenhammar H, et al.: Effects of fasting on disease activity, neutrophil function, fatty acid composition, and leukotriene biosynthesis in patients with rheumatoid arthritis. Arthr Rheum 31:585–92, 1988.

13. De Witte TJ, Geerdink PJ, Lamers CB, et al.: Hypochlorhydria and hypergastrinemia in rheumatoid arthritis. Ann Rheum Dis 38:14–7, 1979.

14. Henriksson K, Uvnas-Moberg K, Nord CE, et al.: Gastrin, gastric acid secretion, and gastric microflora in patients with rheumatoid arthritis. Ann Rheum Dis 45:475–83, 1986.

15. Mojaverian P: Estimation of gastric residence time of the Heidelberg capsule in humans. Gastroenterol 89:392–7, 1985.

16. Wright J: A proposal for standardized challenge testing of gastric acid secretory capacity using the Heidelberg capsule radiotelemetry system. J John Bastyr Col Nat Med 1:2:3–11, 1979.

17. Ambrus JL: Absorption of exogenous and endogenous proteolytic enzymes. Clin Pharmacol Ther 8:362–8, 1967.

18. Avakian, S: Further studies on the absorption of chymotrypsin. Clin Pharmacol Ther 5:712–5, 1964.

19. Liebow C and Rothman SS: Enteropancreatic circulation of digestive enzymes. Science 189:472–4, 1975.

20. Rubinstein E, Mark Z, Haspel J, et al.: Antibacterial activity of the pancreatic fluid. Gastroenterol 88:927–32, 1985.

21. Oelgoetz AW: The treatment of food allergy and indigestion of pancreatic origin with pancreatic enzymes. Am J Dig Dis Nutr 2:422–6, 1935.

22. Innerfield I: Enzymes in Clinical Medicine. McGraw-Hill, New York, 1960.

23. Horger I: Enzyme therapy in multiple rheumatic diseases. Therapiewoche 33:3948–57, 1983.

24. Ransberger K: Enzyme treatment of immune complex diseases. Arthr Rheum 8:16–9, 1986.

25. Steffen C, et al.: Enzyme therapy in comparison with immune complex determinations in chronic polyarteritis. Rheumatologie 44: 51–6, 1985.

26. Ransberger K and van Schaik W: Enzyme therapy in multiple sclerosis. Der Kassenarzt 41:42–5, 1986.

27. Kremer J, Michaelek AV, Lininger L, et al.: Effects of manipulation of dietary fatty acids on clinical manifestation of rheumatoid arthritis. Lancet i:184–7, 1985.

28. Lee TH and Arm JP: Prospects for modifying the allergic response by fish oil diets. Clin Allergy 16:89–100, 1986.

29. Magaro M, Altomonte L, Zoli A, et al.: Influence of diet with different lipid composition on neutrophil composition on neutrophil chemiluminescence and disease activity in patients with rheumatoid arthritis. Ann Rheum Dis 47:793–6, 1988.

30. Darlington LG: Do diets rich in polyunsaturated fatty acids affect disease activity in rheumatoid arthritis? Ann Rheum Dis 47:169–72, 1988.

31. Hansen TM, Lerche A, Kassis V, et al.: Treatment of rheumatoid arthritis with prostaglandin E_1 precursors as cis-linoleic acid and gamma-linolenic acid. Scand J Rheumatol 12:85–8, 1983.

32. Belch JJF, Ansell D, Madhok R, et al.: Effects of altering dietary essential fatty acid on requirements for non-steroidal anti-inflammatory drugs in patients with rheumatoid arthritis: A double-blind placebo-controlled study. Ann Rheum Dis 4:96–104, 1988.

33. Jantti J, Nikkari T, Solakivi T, et al.: Evening primrose oil in rheumatoid arthritis: Changes in serum lipids and fatty acids. Ann Rheum Dis 48:124–7, 1989.

34. Cody V, Middleton E, and Harborne JB: Plant Flavonoids in Biology and Medicine—Biochemical, Pharmacological, and Structure-Activity Relationships. Alan R Liss, New York, 1986.

35. Cody V, Middleton E, Harborne JB, and Beretz A: Plant Flavonoids in Biology and Medicine II—Biochemical, Pharmacological, and Structure-Activity Relationships. Alan R Liss, New York, 1988.

36. Havsteen B: Flavonoids, a class of natural products of high pharmacological potency. Biochemical Pharmacol 32:1141–8, 1983.

37. Kuhnau J: The flavonoids: A class of semi-essential food components: Their role in human nutrition. World R Nutr and Diet 24:117–91, 1976.

38. Blau LW: Cherry diet control for gout and arthritis. Texas Report on Biol and Med 8:309–11, 1950.

39. Middleton E: The flavonoids. Trends in Pharmaceutical Sci 5:335–8, 1984.

40. Tarayre JP and Lauressergues H: Advantages of a combination of proteolytic enzymes, flavonoids and ascorbic acid in comparison with non-steroidal anti-inflammatory agents. Arzneim-Forsch 27: 1144–9, 1977.

41. Tarp U, Overvad K, Hansen JC, et al.: Low selenium level in severe rheumatoid arthritis. Scand J Rheumatol 14:97–101, 1985.

42. Tarp U, Overvad K, Thorling EB, et al.: Selenium treatment in rheumatoid arthritis. Scand J Rheumatol 14:364–8, 1985.

43. Munthe E and Aseth J: Treatment of rheumatoid arthritis with selenium and vitamin E. Scand J Rheumatol 53 (supplement):103, 1984.

44. Pandley SP, Bhattacharya SK, and Sundar S: Zinc in rheumatoid arthritis. Ind J Med Res 81:618–20, 1985.

45. Simkin PA: Treatment of rheumatoid arthritis with oral zinc sulfate. Agents and Actions (supplement) 8:587–95, 1981.

46. Mattingly PC and Mowat AG: Zinc sulphate in rheumatoid arthritis. Ann Rheum Dis 41:456–7, 1982.

47. Pasquier C, Mach PS, Raichvarg D, et al.: Manganese-containing superoxide-dismutase deficiency in polymorphonuclear leukocytes of adults with rheumatoid arthritis. Inflam 8:27–32, 1984.

48. Menander-Huber KB: Orgotein in the treatment of rheumatoid arthritis. Eur J Rheum Inflam 4:201–11, 1981.

49. Zidenberg-Cherr S, Keen CL, Lonnerdal B, et al.: Dietary superoxide dismutase does not affect tissue levels. Am J Clin Nutr 37:5–7, 1983.

50. Rosa GD, Keen CL, Leach RM, et al.: Regulation of superoxide dismutase activity by dietary manganese. J Nutr 110:795–804, 1980.

51. Mullen A and Wilson CWM: The metabolism of ascorbic acid in rheumatoid arthritis. Proc Nutr Sci 35:8A–9A, 1976.

52. Subramanian N: Histamine degradation potential of ascorbic acid. Agents and Actions 8:484–7, 1978.

53. Levine M: New concepts in the biology and biochemistry of ascorbic acid. N Engl J Med 314:892–902, 1986.

54. Barton-Wright EC and Elliott WA: The pantothenic acid metabolism of rheumatoid arthritis. Lancet ii:862–3, 1963.

55. General Practitioner Research Group. Practitioner 224:208–11, 1980.

56. Biemond P, Swaak AG, Eijk HG, et al.: Intraarticular ferritin-bound iron in rheumatoid arthritis. Arthr Rheum 29:1187–93, 1986.

57. Fairbanks VF and Beutler E: Iron. In: Modern Nutrition in Health and Disease, 7th edition. Shils ME and Young VR (eds). Lea and Febiger, Philadelphia, 1988, pp. 193–226.

58. Cazzola P, Mazzanti P, and Bossi G: In vivo modulating effect of a calf thymus acid lysate on human T lymphocyte subsets and CD4+/CD8+ ratio in the course of different diseases. Current Ther Res 42:1011–7, 1987.

59. Kouttab NM, Prada M, and Cazzola P: Thymomodulin: Biological properties and clinical applications. Medical Oncol Tumor Pharmacother 6:5–9, 1989.

60. Ammon HPT and Wahl MA: Pharmacology of *Curcuma longa*. Planta Medica 57:1–7, 1991.

61. Sharma OP: Antioxidant properties of curcumin and related compounds. Biochemical Pharmacol 25:1811–25, 1976.

62. Toda S, Miyase T, Arich H, et al.: Natural antioxidants: Antioxidative compounds isolated from rhizome of *Curcuma longa* L. Chem Pharmacol Bull 33:1725–8, 1985.

63. Srimal R and Dhawan B: Pharmacology of diferuloyl methane (curcumin), a non-steroidal anti-inflammatory agent. J Pharm Pharmac 25:447–52, 1973.

64. Mukhopadhyay A, Basu N, Ghatak N, et al.: Anti-inflammatory and irritant activities of curcumin analogues in rats. Agents and Actions 12:508–15, 1982.

65. Ghatak N and Basu N: Sodium curcuminate as an effective anti-inflammatory agent. Ind J Exp Biol 10:235–6, 1972.

66. Srivastava R and Srimal RC: Modification of certain inflammation-induced biochemical changes by curcumin. Ind J Med Res 81:215–23, 1985.

67. Srivastava R: Inhibition of neutrophil response by curcumin. Agents and Actions 28:298–303, 1989.

68. Flynn DL and Rafferty MF: Inhibition of 5-hydroxy-eicosatetraenoic acid (5-HETE) formation in intact human neutraphils by naturally-occurring diarylheptanoids: Inhibitory activities of curcuminoids and yakuchinones. Prost Leukotri Med 22:357–60, 1986.

69. Deodhar SD, Sethi R, and Srimal RC: Preliminary studies on anti-rheumatic activity of curcumin (diferuloyl methane). Ind J Med Res 71:632–4, 1980.

70. Satoskar RR, Shah SJ, and Shenoy SG: Evaluation of antiinflammatory property of curcumin (diferuloyl methane) in patients with postoperative inflammation. Int J Clin Pharmacol Ther Toxicol 24: 651–4, 1986.

71. Shankar TNB, Shantha NV, Ramesh HP, et al.: Toxicity studies on turmeric (*Curcuma longa*): Acute toxicity studies in rats, guinea pigs & monkeys. Indi J Exp Biol 18:73–5, 1980.

72. Taussig S and Batkin S: Bromelain the enzyme complex of pineapple (*Ananas comosus*) and its clinical application. An update. J Ethnopharmacol 22:191–203, 1988.

73. Cohen A and Goldman J: Bromelain therapy in rheumatoid arthritis. Penn Med J 67:27–30, 1964.

74. Leung A: Encyclopedia of Common Natural Ingredients Used in Food, Drugs, and Cosmetics. Wiley, New York, 1980.

75. Kiuchi F, Iwakami S, Shibuya, et al.: Inhibition of prostaglandin and leukotriene biosynthesis by gingerols and diarylheptanoids. Chem Pharmacol Bull 40:387–91, 1992.

76. Kiuchi F, Shibuyu M, and Sankawa U: Inhibitors of prostaglandin biosynthesis from ginger. Chem Pharmacol Bull 30:754–7, 1982.

77. Srivastava KC and Mustafa T: Ginger (*Zingiber officinale*) and rheumatic disorders. Med Hypothesis 29:25–28, 1989.

78. Srivastava KC and Mustafa T: Ginger (*Zingiber officinale*) in rheumatism and musculoskeletal disorders. Med Hypothesis 39:342–8, 1992.

79. Shimizu K, Amagaya S, and Ogihara Y: Combination of shosaikoto (Chinese traditional medicine) and prednisolone on the anti-inflammatory action. J Pharm Dyn 7:891–9, 1984.

80. Yamamoto M, Kumagai A, and Yokoyama Y: Structure and actions of saikosaponins isolated from *Bupleurum falcatum* L. Arzneim-Forsch 25:1021–40, 1975.

81. Hiai S, Yokoyama H, Nagasawa T, et al.: Stimulation of the pituitary-adrenocortical axis by saikosaponin of *Bupleuri radix*. Chem Pharmacol Bull 29:495–9, 1981.

82. Hikino H: Recent research on Oriental medicinal plants. Econ Med Plant Res 1:53–85, 1985.

83. Sabinsa Corporation: Information on Boswellin. Edison, NJ, 1993.

84. Makheja AM and Bailey JM: A platelet phospholipase inhibitor from the medicinal herb feverfew (*Tanacetum parthenium*). Prost Leukotri Med 8:653–60, 1982.

85. Heptinstall S, White A, Williamson L, et al.: Extracts of feverfew inhibit granule secretion in blood platelets and polymorphonuclear leucocytes. Lancet i:1071–4, 1985.

86. Pattrick M, Heptinstall S, and Doherty M: Feverfew in rheumatoid arthritis: A double blind, placebo controlled study. Ann Rheum Dis 48:547–9, 1989.

87. Johnson ES, Kadam NP, Hylands DM, et al.: Efficacy of feverfew as prophylactic treatment of migraine. Br Med J 291:569–73, 1985.

88. Murphy JJ, Heptinstall S, and Mitchell JRA: Randomized double-blind placebo-controlled trial of feverfew in migraine prevention. Lancet ii:189–92, 1988.

89. Heptinstall S, Awang DVC, Dawson BA, et al.: Parthenolide content and bioactivity of feverfew (*Tanacetum parthenium* (L.) Schultz-Bip.). Estimation of commercial and authenticated feverfew products. J Pharm Pharmac 44:391–5, 1992.

90. Bingham R, Bellew BA, and Bellew JG: Yucca plant saponin in the management of arthritis. J Applied Nutr 27:45–50, 1975.

Chapter 7: The Design of a Healthful Diet

1. Trowell H, Burkitt D, and Heaton K: Dietary Fibre, Fibre-Depleted Foods and Disease. Academic Press, New York, 1985.

2. US Dept of Health and Human Services: The Surgeon General's Report on Nutrition and Health. Prima, Rocklin, CA, 1988.

3. National Research Council: Diet and Health. Implications for Reducing Chronic Disease Risk. National Academy Press, Washington, D.C., 1989.

4. Murray MT and Pizzorno JE: Encyclopedia of Natural Medicine. Prima, Rocklin, CA, 1991.

5. Brostoff J and Challacombe SJ (eds): Food Allergy and Intolerance. Saunders, Philadelphia, 1987.

6. Kjeldsen-Kragh J, Haugen M, Borchgrevink CF, et al.: Controlled trial of fasting and one-year vegetarian diet in rheumatoid arthritis. Lancet 338:899–902, 1991.

Index

diets of, 105–110
fats and oils in, 117–119
food allergies and, 127–131
fruits in, 113–114
legumes in, 116–117
meat, fish, cheese, and eggs
  in, 120–121
menu planning in, 121–122
milk in, 119
starchy vegetables in,
  114–116
vegetables in, 110–112
Heart disease, 10
Heart inflammation, 46
Heidelberg gastric analysis,
  60
Heme iron, 80–81
Hepatitis B infections, 82
Herring, 38
Histamine, 52, 127
Hydrochloric acid, 59, 60
  dosage of, 61
Hydroxychloroquine, 53
Hypochlorhydria, 60

I

Ibuprofen, 6
  glucosamine sulfate
    compared to, 13–14
Ideal body weight, 103–105
IgE antibodies, 127
Immune complexes, 48–49
  proteases and, 64–65
Indocin, 6
Indometh, 6
Indomethacin, 6, 32
Inflammatory mediators, 51–52
Iron and rheumatoid arthritis,
  80–81
Isometric exercises for
  osteoarthritis, 22

J

Juicers, 11

K

Kaufman, William, 18
Kidneys
  damage to, 7
  fluid intake and stones, 39
  gout and, 29
Kinins, 86
Korean ginseng root, 89–90

L

Lactate production, 38
The Lancet, 55
Lead toxicity and gout, 41–42
Legumes
  in Healthy Exchange System,
    116–117
  lead and, 42
Leukotrienes, 52, 66
  curcumin and, 84
Licorice, deglycyrrhizinated
    (DGL), 23–24
Licorice root, 20, 89–90
Linoleic acid, 68
  conversion to
    prostaglandins, 69
Linolenic acid, 69
Lipase, 65
Liquid Liver Extract, Enzymatic
    Therapy, 81
Liver
  damage to, 7
  licorice and, 89
  Liquid Liver Extract,
    Enzymatic Therapy, 81
Low gastric acidity, 60–61
Low-purine diet, 38
Lunch recipes, 123–125
Lung inflammation, 46

for gout, 40
Omega-3 prostaglandin
    pathway, 70–79
Omega-6 oils, 68–69
Omnivore diets
    1,500-calorie omnivore diet,
        107
    2,000-calorie omnivore diet,
        108
    2,500-calorie omnivore diet,
        108–109
    3,000-calorie omnivore diet,
        109–110
Onions, 11
Oral supplements. *See*
    Nutritional supplements
Organ meats, 27, 38
Oslo Rheumatism Hospital
    study, 58–59
Osteoarthritis, 3–26
    current medical treatment
        of, 6–8
    signs of, 4

P

Panax ginseng, 89–90
Pancreas, 60. *See also*
    Proteases
Pancreatic enzymes, 59, 62–63
    dosage of, 66
Pancreatin, 65
    dosage of, 66
Pantothenic acid, 12
    for osteoarthritis, 18
    for rheumatoid arthritis, 80
Papin, 65
Parthenolide content of
    feverfew products, 91
Pauling, Linus, 17
Penicillamine, 54
Peppers, 12

Peptic ulcers, 7
Periarteritis nodos, 64
Pesticides, 10
Phenylbutazone, 32
pH level of stomach, 60
Physical exercises. *See*
    Exercises
Physical therapy
    for osteoarthritis, 22
    for rheumatoid arthritis,
        93
Phytoestrogens, 20
Pineapple-ginger juice, 87
Piroxicam, 7
Plant-based medicines
    for gout, 41
    for osteoarthritis, 19–21
    for rheumatoid arthritis,
        83–93
Plaquenil, 53
Potatoes, 12
Prednisolone, 51
Prednisone, 51–52
Primary gout, 29–30
Primary osteoarthritis, 4–5
Proanthocyanidins, 39, 74
Proben-C, 33
Probenecid, 33, 34–35
Pro-oxidants, 10
Prostaglandins, 52, 66
    linoleic and linolenic acids
        and, 69
    omega-3 prostaglandin
        pathway, 70–79
Proteases, 62
    dosage of, 66
    importance of, 63–65
Protein
    and gout, 38–39
    in Healthy Exchange System,
        101

2,500-calorie vegan diet, 109

U

Ulcerative colitis. *See* Colitis
Ulcers, 7
  DGL for, 23–24
United States Pharmacopeia
    (USP), 66
Unsaturated fats, 67
Uric acid, 30–31

V

Vasculitis, 46
Vegan diet
  arachidonic acid and, 69
Vegan diets
  1,500-calorie vegan diet,
      106–107
  2,000-calorie vegan diet, 107
  2,500-calorie vegan diet, 109
  3,000-calorie vegan diet, 109
Vegetables in Healthy
    Exchange System,
    110–112
Vitamin A, 18–19
Vitamin B3, 18
Vitamin B5, 12, 18
Vitamin B6, 12, 18–19
Vitamin B12, 41
Vitamin C, 11, 12, 16–17
  lead and, 42
  and rheumatoid arthritis, 79
  smoking and, 10

Vitamin E, 10, 11, 12, 16–17
  and rheumatoid arthritis,
      77–78

W

Weight
  gout and obesity, 38
  ideal body weight, 103–105
Wheat allergy, 130
Whole grains, lead and, 42

X

Xanthine oxidase, 40
X rays, 10

Y

Yeast, 38
Yucca aborescens, 92–93
Yucca for rheumatoid arthritis,
    92–93

Z

Zantac, 23–24
Zinc, 12
  and osteoarthritis, 18–19
  and rheumatoid arthritis, 78
Zinc citrate, 78
Zinc monomethionine, 78
Zinc picolinate, 78
Zingiber officinale, 87

Vital Communications

Natural Medicine Update

So much is happening in health and healing, it's almost impossible to keep up to date. That's why each month Dr. Murray writes "Vital Communications: Natural Medicine Update"—to keep you informed on the medical breakthroughs that can give you the health you deserve. Each issue is packed full of practical information that you can put to use. Answers are provided to even the most difficult health questions.

- Discover vital health secrets.
- Learn the latest in nutrition and herb research.
- Stay informed and up to date.

For a free issue of "Vital Communications," write or call:

Vital Communications
15401 S.E. 54th Ct.
Bellevue, WA 98006
1-800-488-0753

Diabetes and hypoglycemia, the major causes of blood sugar imbalance, are the most common of all diseases and can lead to chronic metabolic problems. Often traditional medications treat only specific symptoms without treating the whole body. Here, Dr. Murray offers the answers you need in chapters such as:

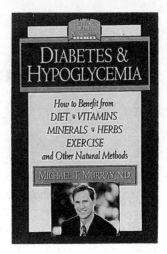

- early symptoms and proper diagnosis
- herbal remedies
- essential vitamins for blood sugar control
- plants as means of blood sugar control

Chronic fatigue syndrome is a widespread phenomenon, and society has just recently recognized its seriousness. Because many sufferers prefer not to use heavy doses of medication to treat symptoms, Dr. Murray offers natural, alternative treatments. He covers subjects such as:

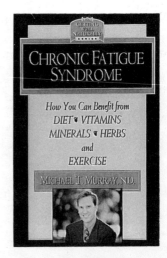

- diagnosing chronic fatigue syndrome
- plant-based medicines for chronic fatigue
- the energy prescription
- chronic fatigue and the liver, adrenal, and immune functions

Menopause is a natural part of life, and the way you deal with it should be too. Dr. Michael Murray, one of the world's foremost authorities in nutritional and natural medicine, presents a natural approach to deal with the effects of menopause. He covers topics such as:

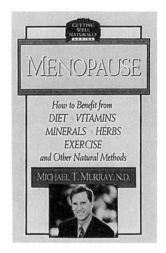

- the causes of menopause
- the benefits and risks of estrogen replacement therapy
- herbal remedies and natural foods that can control symptoms
- vitamins and minerals to enhance circulation

Your sexual vitality is important to you and to the one you love. It encompasses both performance and fertility and affects the way you feel about yourself. In *Male Sexual Vitality*, Dr. Michael Murray suggests a natural approach to regaining and maintaining your energy. He covers topics such as:

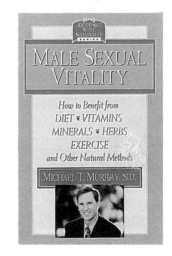

- specific nutrients for optimal sexual function
- understanding impotence
- causes and treatments for low sperm count
- natural herbs for enhanced libido and performance—regardless of age

FILL IN AND MAIL TODAY

PRIMA PUBLISHING
P.O. BOX 1260BK
ROCKLIN, CA 95677

USE YOUR VISA/MC AND ORDER BY PHONE:
(916) 632-4400 (M-F 9:00-4:00 PST)

Please send me the following titles:

Quantity	Title	Amount
_____	_____	_____
_____	_____	_____
_____	_____	_____
_____	_____	_____
_____	_____	_____

Subtotal $_____

Postage & Handling
($4.00 for the first book
plus $1.00 each additional book) $ _____

Sales Tax
7.25% Sales Tax (California only)
8.25% Sales Tax (Tennessee only)
5.00% Sales Tax (Maryland only)
7.00% General Service Tax (Canada) $_____

TOTAL *(U.S. funds only)* $_____

❏ Check enclosed for $_____(payable to Prima Publishing)

Charge my   ❏ Master Card   ❏ Visa

Account No. _____Exp. Date _____

Signature _____

Your Name _____

Address _____

City/State/Zip _____

Daytime Telephone _____

Satisfaction is guaranteed— or your money back!
Please allow three to four weeks for delivery.
THANK YOU FOR YOUR ORDER